The
Hypothalamic-Pituitary-Adrenal Axis

Physiology, Pathophysiology, and Psychiatric Implications

The Hypothalamic-Pituitary-Adrenal Axis

Physiology, Pathophysiology, and Psychiatric Implications

Editors

Alan F. Schatzberg, M.D.

Service Chief and Director,
Depression Research Facility
McLean Hospital
Associate Professor of Psychiatry
Harvard Medical School
Boston, Massachusetts

Charles B. Nemeroff, M.D., Ph.D.

Director, Laboratory of Psychoneuroendocrinology
Associate Professor of Psychiatry and Pharmacology
Duke University Medical Center
Durham, North Carolina

Raven Press 🖹 New York

Raven Press, 1185 Avenue of the Americas, New York, New York 10036

Made in the United States of America

Library of Congress Cataloging-in-Publication Data

The Hypothalamic-pituitary-adrenal axis : physiology, pathophysiology, and psychiatric implications / editors, Alan F. Schatzberg, Charles B. Nemeroff.
    p. cm.
  Updated papers presented at a symposium held at the annual meeting of the American College of Neuropsychopharmacology in Maui, Hawaii, Dec. 1985.
  Includes bibliographies and index.
  ISBN 0-88167-393-5
  1. Hypothalamic-pituitary-adrenal axis—Congresses.
2. Hypothalamic-pituitary-adrenal axis—Pathophysiology—Congresses.
3. Depression, Mental—Pathophysiology—Congresses. I. Schatzberg, Alan F. II. Nemeroff, Charles B. III. American College of Neuropsychopharmacology. Meeting (24th : 1985 : Maui, Hawaii)
  [DNLM: 1. Corticotropin Releasing Hormone—physiology—congresses.
2. Depressive Disorder—physiopathology—congresses. 3. Hypothalamo -Hypophyseal System—physiopathology—congresses. 4. Pituitary -Adrenal System—physiopathology—congresses. WK 510 H998]
QP188.H88H97 1988
616.85'27071—dc19
DNLM/DLC   87-35966
for Library of Congress   CIP

9 8 7 6 5 4 3 2 1

*To our wives and children who have so patiently put up
with our long hours at work and away from home*

Preface

Over the past two decades, the activity of the HPA axis has frequently been the focus of much research in psychiatry. Various approaches have been taken over the past 20 years, in part reflecting then current theoretical thinking and available technology. Early studies emphasized the markedly elevated 24-hour urinary 17-hydroxy-corticosteroid concentrations observed in various psychiatric patients. Often cortisol hypersecretion was viewed as reflecting the degree of patients' ego disintegration, severity of illness, or exposure to stress. The advent of radioimmunoassay (RIA) techniques allowed not only for the precise determination of cortisol in plasma or serum, but also for the study of circadian rhythms in man. These approaches pointed to a marked disruption of the HPA axis in severe endogenous-type depressive disorders as evidenced by increased frequency and amplitude of secretory episodes. These studies were quickly coupled with the application of the dexamethasone suppression test (DST)—in psychiatry—response to a challenge with 1 or 2 mg. dexamethasone, a synthetic glucocorticoid that suppresses cortisol secretion on healthy individuals. In the past 5 or 6 years, the DST has attracted considerable interest and debate—as a potentially specific test for endogenous or melancholic depressive disorders.

Challenges with dexamethasone were also used to explore the neurochemical control of the HPA axis. Acetylcholine and serotonin have generally been thought to stimulate cortisol secretion, probably by stimulating secretion of corticotropin releasing factor (CRF), a neuropeptide whose structure has only recently been identified. (In contrast, early studies suggested norepinephrine inhibited CRF, although more recent studies have brought this into question.) In this overall approach, HPA disruption was viewed as a window to understanding the neurotransmitter basis of depressive disorders. A variety of strategies that employed stimulation of those neurotransmitters that controlled cortisol secretion (e.g., serotonin, acetylcholine, and norepinephrine) were developed to test these hypotheses.

The eventual identification of the amino acid sequence of CRF led to further changes in the approaches to studying HPA physiology. CRF could now be infused into patients to study patterns of adrenocorticotropin (ACTH) and cortisol response in patients and controls. Moreover, CRF could be measured in both postmortem brain tissue and cerebrospinal fluid. Coupling studies in man with those in lower animal species, investigators have more recently begun to posit that CRF itself was a neurotransmitter/neuromodulator, and that could itself cause behavioral disturbances, including depression. In addition, studies from a number of groups have suggested that cortisol itself could be "toxic," leading to psychosis, loss of hippocampal neurons, etc. Thus, in more recent years, the HPA axis has become viewed as a key party in the expression of psychiatric disturbances rather than as a mere window to the brain. Such approaches offer additional opportunities for developing new theories as to the biological underpinnings of various psychiatric syndromes, particularly depression.

The excitement of this research and of these newer approaches is captured in the various chapters in this book. In addition, the fundamental basis of HPA physiology/pathophysiology is also reviewed to allow the reader to develop a comprehensive understanding of this important system.

Alan F. Schatzberg
Charles B. Nemeroff

Acknowledgments

In December, 1985, a symposium was held at the annual meeting of the American College of Neuropsychopharmacology (ACNP) in Maui, Hawaii. This symposium, organized and chaired by the editors, gathered a number of investigators to discuss their research on the hypothalamic-pituitary-adrenal (HPA) axis. Evident that day were the great strides that have been made in recent years in understanding the central role this system plays in both the expression and pathophysiology of psychiatric disorders. That excitement served as the impetus to edit this volume which consists primarily of chapters by presenters at that symposium. Because of the rapid evolution of this field, contributors have included in their chapters new data, beyond those presented at the ACNP symposium. We wish to thank all the authors for their contributions, and also to express our appreciation to the American College of Neuropsychopharmacology for including this symposium in their program.

This work was supported in part by NIMH grants MH38671 (AFS), MH42088 (CBN), MH40159 (CBN), and MH40524 (CBN); a grant from the Engelhard Foundation (AFS); and an anonymous gift to the McLean Hospital Depression Research Facility (AFS).

Mrs. Linda Messier Dent assisted in the preparation of the manuscript.

Contents

Contributors

Ulrich von Bardeleben, M.D.
Klinikum der Johannes Gutenberg
Universitat
Postfach 3960
6500 Mainz, Langenbeckstrasse 1
West Germany

Harry A. Brandt, M.D.
Department of Health and Human
Services
National Institute of Mental Health
National Institutes of Health
Bethesda, Maryland 20205

Karen T. Britton, M.D., Ph.D.
Scripps Clinic
10666 North Torrey Pines Road
La Jolla, California 92037

Bernard J. Carroll, M.D., Ph.D.
Duke University Medical Center
Box 3950
Durham, North Carolina 27710

George P. Chrouses, M.D.
Department of Health and Human
Services
National Institute of Mental Health
National Institutes of Health
Bethesda, Maryland 20205

Mark A. Demitrack, M.D.
Department of Health and Human
Services
National Institute of Mental Health
National Institutes of Health
Bethesda, Maryland 20205

Dwight L. Evans, M.D.
Department of Psychiatry
School of Medicine
University of North Carolina
Chapel Hill, North Carolina 27514

Randal D. France, M.D.
Duke University Medical Center
Box 3903
Durham, North Carolina 27710

J. Christian Gillin, M.D.
Department of Psychiatry
M-003
University of California, San Diego
La Jolla, California 92093

Philip W. Gold, M.D.
Department of Health and Human
Services
National Institute of Mental Health
National Institutes of Health
Bethesda, Maryland 20205

Isabella Heuser, M.D.
Klinikum der Johannes Gutenberg
Universitat
Postfach 3960
6500 Mainz, Langenbeckstrasse 1
West Germany

Florien Holsboer, M.D., Ph.D.
Klinikum der Johannes Gutenberg
Universitat
Postfach 3960
6500 Mainz, Langenbeckstrasse 1
West Germany

Leighton Huey, M.D.
Department of Psychiatry
M-003
University of California, San Diego
La Jolla, California 92093

David S. Janowsky, M.D.
Department of Psychiatry
School of Medicine
University of North Carolina
Chapel Hill, North Carolina 27514

Karen L. Johnson
Duke University Medical Center
Box 3870
Durham, North Carolina 27710

Lewis Judd, M.D.
Department of Psychiatry
M-003
University of California, San Diego
La Jolla, California 92093

Ned H. Kalin, M.D.
University of Wisconsin Medical
* School*
Department of Psychiatry
600 Highland Avenue
Madison, Wisconsin 53729

Clinton Kilts, Ph.D.
Duke University Medical Center
Box 3870
Durham, North Carolina 27710

Mitchel A. Kling, M.D.
Department of Health and Human
* Services*
National Institute of Mental Health
National Institutes of Health
Bethesda, Maryland 20205

George F. Koob, Ph.D.
Scripps Clinic
10666 North Torrey Pines Road
La Jolla, California 92037

K. Ranga Rama Krishnan, M.D.
Duke University Medical Center
Box 3215
Durham, North Carolina 27710

Ananth N. Manepalli, M.D.
Duke University Medical Center
Box 2859
Dorham, North Carolina 27710

Bruce S. McEwen, Ph.D.
The Rockefeller University
1230 York Avenue
New York, New York 10021-6399

Miriam A. Mott
Department of Psychiatry
M—003
University of California, San Diego
La Jolla, California 92093

Charles B. Nemeroff, MD., Ph.D.
Duke University Medical Center
Box 2859
Durham, North Carolina 27710

Michael J. Owens
Duke University Medical Center
Box 2859
Durham, North Carolina 27710

Jeffrey L. Rausch, M.D.
Department of Psychiatry
M-003
University of California, San Diego
La Jolla, California 92093

S. Craig Risch, M.D.
Department of Psychiatry
M-003
University of California, San Diego
La Jolla, California 92093

James C. Ritchie, M.P.H.
Duke University Medical Center
Box 2859
Durham, North Carolina 27710

Anthony J. Rothschild, M.D.
McLean Hospital
115 Mill Street
Belmont, Massachusetts 02178

Alan F. Schatzberg, M.D.
McLean Hospital
115 Mill Street
Belmont, Massachusetts 02178

Robert M. Sopolsky, Ph.D.
Department of Biological Sciences
Stanford University
Stanford, California 94305

Axel Steiger, M.D.
Klinikum der Johannes Gutenberg
  Universitat
Postfach 3960
6500 Mainz, Langenbeckstrasse 1
West Germany

Lorey K. Takahashi, Ph.D.
University of Wisconsin Medical
  School
Department of Psychiatry
600 Highland Avenue
Madison, Wisconsin 53729

Sanjeev Venkataraman, M.D.
Duke University Medical Center
Box 2859
Durham, North Carolina 27710

Harvey J. Whitfield, M.D.
Department of Health and Human
  Services
National Institute of Mental Health
National Institutes of Health
Bethesda, Maryland 20205

The
Hypothalamic-Pituitary-Adrenal
Axis

Physiology, Pathophysiology, and Psychiatric Implications

The Hypothalamic-Pituitary-Adrenal Axis:
Physiology, Pathophysiology, and Psychiatric
Implications, edited by A.F. Schatzberg and
C.B. Nemeroff. Raven Press, Ltd., New York
© 1988.

THE NEUROBIOLOGY OF CORTICOTROPIN-RELEASING FACTOR:

IMPLICATIONS FOR AFFECTIVE DISORDERS

Michael J. Owens and Charles B. Nemeroff

Departments of Pharmacology and Psychiatry
Duke University Medical Center
Durham, North Carolina 27710

INTRODUCTION

Elucidation of the chemical identity of corticotropin-releasing factor (CRF) was clearly of paramount importance to any comprehensive understanding of the neural mechanisms that mediate the hypothalamic-pituitary-adrenal (HPA) response to stress. The clinical importance of the HPA axis, and the availability of bioassays for ACTH led investigators in the early 1950's to focus on CRF before investigations of other putative hypothalamic releasing factors. Characterization of CRF proved difficult for several reasons. First, the ease with which almost any novel stimulus (mild stressor) activates the HPA axis in experimental animals has confounded many studies. Secondly, because several drugs and tissue extracts other than CRF can enhance ACTH secretion, e.g., vasopressin, extreme caution was necessary before any endogenous substance could be deemed the physiological CRF. This was a particular problem in regard to the bioassay used to identify CRF activity, i.e., a bioassay for ACTH release from hemipituitaries in vitro. The radioimmunoassay for ACTH also proved to be problematic.

The systemic search for CRF in hypothalamic tissue began with the work of Saffran and Schally [211] and Guillemin and Rosenberg [87]. Subsequently, Schally and Guillemin worked together at McGill University and, using extracts of neurohypophysial tissue and gel filtration chromatography, they discovered CRF activity in three separate fractions which they labeled α-1, α-2 (similar to α-MSH) and β (similar to vasopressin) [219, 220]. Guillemin et al. [88] also discovered that extracts of pig hypothalamus contained ACTH and α- and β-MSH, and although remarkable in that it anticipated by sixteen years the discovery of POMC derived peptides in the brain [129], this finding further increased the difficulty of interpreting the assay data, and serious work on the isolation of CRF was brought to a halt [67].

As alluded to above, the more than 25 year delay in the characterization of CRF after evidence for its existence was unequivocal can be attributed to several factors. The bioassays were problematic because of their lack of specificity, though their sensitivity was often remarkable. Interpretation of even the best in vitro assays could be confounded by the fact that numerous substances, e.g. vasopressin, oxytocin and epinephrine release ACTH and potentiate the effects of CRF. Furthermore, most hypothalamic extracts contain ACTH. In addition, because the sizes of CRF (41 amino acids) and ACTH (39 amino acids) are similar, the two peptides are not easily separated by classical liquid chromatography. In vitro bioassay systems are also vulnerable to nonspecific secretagogues found in tissue extracts such as myelin basic protein, histones, potassium and the components of various buffers and solvents [256].

In 1981, Vale et al. isolated and characterized a 41 amino acid peptide from extracts of ovine hypothalamus with the following primary structure: H-Ser-Gln-Glu-Pro-Pro-Ile-Ser-Leu-Asp-Leu-Thr-Phe-His-Leu-Leu-Arg-Glu-Val-Leu-Glu-Met-Thr-Lys-Ala-Asp-Gln-Leu-Ala-Gln-Gln-Ala-His-Ser-Asn-Arg-Lys-Leu-Leu-Asp-Ile-Ala-NH$_2$ [255, 235]. Starting material for this purification was a side fraction of 490,000 fragments of ovine hypothalamus (initially processed for the characterization of luteinizing hormone-releasing hormone [LH-RH]).

The structure of ovine CRF (oCRF) is homologous with several known peptides including sauvagine and urotensin I. Sauvagine was isolated from the skin of the South American frog Phylomedusa sauvagei. Over 50% of the residues in sauvagine are identical to those in oCRF; the majority remaining are conservative substitutions. Both sauvagine and oCRF are closely related to a third peptide, urotensin I, isolated from the urohypophysis of two species of fish. CRF also shows some homology with calmodulin and with angiotensinogen. The tetrapeptide Phe-His-Leu-Leu is common to both angiotensinogen and oCRF and is the site in angiotensinogen of renin and converting enzyme cleavage. This may reflect a distant ancestral relationship between angiotensinogen and oCRF, each of which can modulate adrenocortical function [256].

Rat and human CRF have an identical structure and differ from oCRF in only seven of the 41 residues. Recently, Schally's group has isolated a 41 amino acid peptide thought to represent the major porcine CRF. This peptide differs from rat/human CRF in only the two N-terminal amino acids [166]. Numa et al. [227, 70] have cloned the DNA sequences complimentary to the human and ovine mRNA encoding for the CRF precursor (prepro-CRF). Comparison of the amino acid sequence of ovine prepro-CRF with that of the ACTH- -LPH precursor and the AVP-neurophysin II precursor suggest that these precursor proteins may be evolutionarily related.

Lau [130] has described the physiochemical properties of CRF. The peptide forms a random coil in aqueous solution. At concentrations greater than 1 uM, the peptide has a tendency to self aggregate. CRF also forms an insoluble monolayer at the air-water interface. These observations and others suggest that the binding of CRF to the membrane receptor is accompanied by the induction of an -helical secondary structure. The -helix formed by this molecule is highly amphiphilic - i.e., the hydrophilic and hydrophobic regions are segregated on opposite faces of the helix. Several modified, amino-terminal shortened CRF fragments have been found to possess CRF antagonist properties both in vivo and in vitro, -helical CRF$_{9-41}$ being commercially available [197].

Localization of CRF

Immunohistochemical methods have been used to visualize CRF-containing fibers and perikarya in the mammalian central nervous system (CNS). Cell bodies that stain positively for immunoreactive CRF are located heterogeneously in many brain regions (Figure 1). The most widely recognized and intensively studied population of CRF neurons are located in the parvocellular region of the paraventricular nucleus (PVN). Their major projection is to the median eminence of the hypothalamus, the site of the primary plexus of the hypothalamo-hypophyseal portal system [8, 217, 143, 174, 133, 46]. Staining in the PVN increases following colchicine treatment and adrenalectomy in rats [7]. Several reports have demonstrated CRF-containing cell bodies in various other hypothalamic nuclei and these appear to contribute to the CRF projections to the median eminence as well. These CRF positive cell bodies have been observed in the supraoptic, suprachiasmatic, preoptic, premammillary, periventricular and arcuate nuclei [47, 48, 216, 144]. Fibers with CRF immunoreactivity have been observed emanating from the PVN, periventricular and supraoptic nuclei and coursing towards the bed nucleus of the stria terminalis, as well as to the median eminence [125]. A second collection of CRF cell bodies has been reported in the central and medial nuclei of the amygdala [66, 147, 125] which is known to project to the hypothalamus, bed nucleus of the stria terminalis, and the parabrachial nucleus. A third population of cell bodies staining positively for CRF arises in scattered cells in the anterior hypothalamus and continues as a wide band of concentrated cells through the preoptic area/diagonal band/septal region and projects to the nucleus accumbens and the olfactory tubercles [172]. Classical neuroanatomical methods have revealed that the stria terminalis receives projections from many of these neurons, but their ultimate destination is largely unknown. A fourth group of CRF cell bodies is found in the parabrachial nucleus of the pons and the adjacent locus coeruleus (LC) [218]; it sends fibers posteriorly to the medulla as well as rostrally towards the lateral hypothalamus. A high density of CRF-positive staining is seen in the molecular layer of the temporal cortex, globus pallidus and inferior olive. Definite, but significantly less dense fiber staining is observed in the molecular layer of the subiculum and cingulate cortex [125].

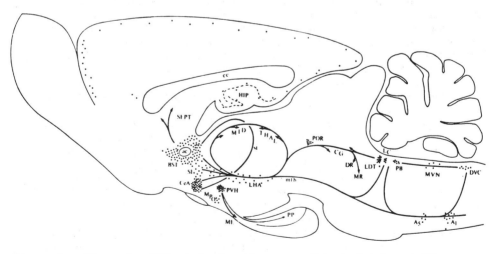

Figure 1. The major CRF-stained cell groups (black dots) and fiber systems are illustrated schematically in this sagittal view of the rat brain. Most of the immunoreactive cells and fibers appear to be associated with systems that regulate the output of the pituitary and

the autonomic nervous system, and with cortical interneurons. Most of
the longer central fibers course either ventrally through the medial
forebrain bundle and its caudal extension in the reticular formation,
or dorsally through a periventricular system in the thalamus and brain
stem central gray. The direction of fibers in these systems is unclear
because they appear to interconnect regions that contain CRF-stained
cell bodies. Thus, for example, three adjacent CRF-stained cell
groups, the laterodorsal tegmental nucleus (LDT), LC, and parabrachial
nucleus (PB), lie in the dorsal pons. However, it is uncertain which
of these cell groups contributes to each of the pathways shown, and
which of them receives inputs from the same pathways. Taken from
Swanson [244].

   Using the micropunch dissection techniques of Palkovits [165] coupled
with a sensitive and specific radioimmunoassay to measure CRF, our
group [122, 40] has determined the distribution of CRF in 32 individual
rat brain nuclei. We found measurable concentrations of CRF in all of
the brain areas studied (Table 1).
   This heterogenous distribution of CRF is concordant with a role for
the peptide as a neurotransmitter or neuromodulator in the CNS. The
distribution of immunoreactive CRF generally parallels the pattern
demonstrated for CRF fibers and cell bodies as visualized by
immunohistochemical techniques.
   Functional roles for chemical messengers in the CNS can, to some
extent, be inferred from neuroanatomic localization. Thus consistent
with a role for CRF as a hypothalamic-releasing factor regulating
pituitary-adrenal activity is the presence of CRF in high concentrations in the PVN and the median eminence the so called hypophysiotropic
areas of the hypothalamus. Relatively high concentrations of CRF have,
as noted above, been discovered in subcortical limbic and brain stem
structures (e.g., amygdala, bed nucleus of the stria terminalis, raphe
nuclei), brain regions traditionally associated with control of a
variety of behaviors and affect. Furthermore, considerable variance in
the concentrations of CRF was observed among the component nuclei of
the amygdala and hypothalamus, suggesting that the functional role of
CRF would most likely vary among these individual nuclei. High
concentrations of CRF were also noted in brain regions containing major
perikarya for the catecholamine (norepinephrine and dopamine) and
indoleamine (serotonin) neurotransmitters. Thus, CRF is strategically
positioned to influence the activity of the major monoamine-containing
neuronal systems in the CNS.
   Although perhaps not directly pertinent to the current discussion, it
is important to note that several investigators have observed
CRF-containing cells in the periphery. In the pancreas, CRF immunoreactive cells are scattered throughout the endocrine pancreas in a
pattern similar to the glucagon-containing A cells. Immunoreactive CRF
has also been found in the stomach and small intestine [171, 170]. In
addition, CRF has also been reported in the adrenal medulla and cortex,
certain lung carcinomas and pheochromocytomas [237]. Bruhn [28] has
demonstrated a releasable pool of CRF from the dog adrenal medulla that
may act locally within the gland as a paracrine substance. CRF has
also been detected in plasma of women in their third trimester of
pregnancy, the source of which is probably the placenta [214].
   Investigators over the past several years have unequivocally demonstrated that several chemical messengers may be colocalized within the

TABLE 1. Concentration of CRF-Like Immunoreactivity (CRF-LI) in
Discrete Microdissected Nuclei of the Rat Brain

Brain Region	n	pg CRF-LI/mg protein
		mean $\pm$ SEM
Hypothalamic nuclei		
Paraventricular	10	498 $\pm$ 44
Periventricular	10	316 $\pm$ 15
Arcuate/Median eminence	8	5054 $\pm$ 674
Anterior	10	93 $\pm$ 7
Dorsomedial	8	114 $\pm$ 7
Ventromedial	10	97 $\pm$ 15
Medial preoptic	9	143 $\pm$ 11
Lateral preoptic	10	86 $\pm$ 6
Interstitial (bed) nucleus of the		
stria terminalis	10	136 $\pm$ 14
Amygdaloid nuclei		
Central	10	192 $\pm$ 17
Lateral	9	77 $\pm$ 5
Basal	10	85 $\pm$ 3
Medial	10	110 $\pm$ 10
Cortical	8	129 $\pm$ 9
Nucleus accumbens	10	94 $\pm$ 12
Olfactory tubercle	10	94 $\pm$ 7
Brainstem nuclei		
Ventral tegmental area	8	134 $\pm$ 11
Substantia nigra pars compacta	10	190 $\pm$ 13
Substantia nigra pars reticulata	10	94 $\pm$ 7
Locus coeruleus	10	148 $\pm$ 9
Dorsal raphe	8	236 $\pm$ 28
Medial raphe	10	241 $\pm$ 19
Dorsal motor complex	10	194 $\pm$ 15
Periaqueductal gray	10	144 $\pm$ 18
Septal nuclei		
Lateral	10	68 $\pm$ 7
Medial	10	86 $\pm$ 9
Hippocampus		
Dorsal	10	31 $\pm$ 2
Ventral	10	35 $\pm$ 2
Cerebrocortical areas		
Entorhinal	10	27 $\pm$ 3
Cingulate	10	12 $\pm$ 1.7
Medial prefrontal	10	22 $\pm$ 1
Piriform	10	28 $\pm$ 1.8

[n] number of replications per brain region.

same neurons. This has now been demonstrated for CRF. A number of oxytocin-staining cells in the magnocellular division of the supraoptic and PVN of the hypothalamus also stain positively for CRF. Moreover, smaller numbers of neurotensin-containing and vasopressin-containing cells in the parvocellular division of the PVN also contain CRF-like immunoreactivity [216]. It has been reported that 44% of the CRF-containing nerve terminals in the median eminence also stain for vasopressin; this is increased to nearly 100% after adrenalectomy [264]. Although not demonstrable in intact animals, CRF and vasopressin have been shown to be colocalized in the parvocellular perikarya of the PVN following adrenalectomy [175]. CRF has also been shown to be colocalized with dynorphin-(1-8), enkephalin and PHI 1-27 in the PVN [209, 103]. Co-localization of substance P, CRF and acetylcholinesterase has been detected by retrograde tracing and immunocytochemical staining in a midbrain projection to the medial prefrontal cortex, septum and thalamus of the rat [43]. Furthermore, CRF immunoreactivity has been reported to be colocalized with substance P, somatostatin and leu-enkephalin in the dorsal root and trigeminal ganglia, laminae I and II of the dorsal horn of the spinal cord, substantia gelatinosa, lateral border of the spinal nucleus and in the tractus spinalis of the trigeminal nerve [231].

Receptors for CRF

Using both autoradiographic and biochemical methods, the highest concentrations of CRF binding sites, putative CRF receptors, in the rat are found in the anterior and intermediate lobes of the pituitary. High concentrations of CRF binding sites are also found in the olfactory bulb, cerebellum, layers I and IV of the neocortex, striatum and amygdala. Moderate to high densities of CRF binding are found in the PVN and the median eminence. These latter binding sites may represent presynaptic autoreceptors. Progressively lower, but detectable, concentrations of CRF binding sites occur in other hypothalamic nuclei, as well as in parts of the medulla, midbrain, pons, thalamus, hippocampus and cervical spinal cord [56, 51, 52, 55, 146, 269]. In general those brain areas high in CRF receptor sites are well correlated with areas containing high endogenous concentrations of CRF-LI. The cerebellum and olfactory bulb are, however, two major exceptions. Although the cerebellum and olfactory bulb contain a high density of CRF binding sites, there is little immunoreactive CRF present in these regions. These may represent nonfunctional receptors conserved during the evolutionary process. However, a recent report [184] suggests a functional CRF pathway from the inferior olive complex to the cerebellum. This problem of "mismatches" has been noted in previous studies involving both classical neurotransmitters and neuropeptides [97].

Adrenalectomized animals exhibit a decrease in the number of adenohypophyseal binding sites for CRF; no changes were observed in any other brain regions [54, 268]. This receptor down-regulation is most likely due to the increased CRF release in response to the lack of glucocorticoid feedback. While it has been shown that this decrease in binding can be reversed by dexamethasone [54, 268], recently chronic corticosterone administration has been reported to decrease CRF binding in the pituitary, without any alterations in other brain regions [93].

Binding sites for CRF have also been described in the periphery. The CRF binding sites in primate adrenal medulla are coupled to adenylate cyclase and their activation results in catecholamine and met-enkephalin secretion [251]. Saturation studies of the CRF receptors in adrenal membranes and bovine chromaffin cells reveals the existence of both low and high affinity binding sites [49]. Putative CRF receptors have also been identified in sympathetic ganglia, kidney, ureter, urinary bladder and erythrocytes, but not lymphocytes [251, 50].

A fluorescent analog of the peptide (fluorescein-Ser[1], Nle[21,39] Arg[36]) rCRF has recently been synthesized. It should prove useful in visualizing cells containing CRF receptors [224].

These high affinity specific binding sites for CRF exhibit time and temperature dependency, sensitivity to pH changes, as well as to ionic strength and cationic composition. As noted above putative CRF receptors are known to be coupled to adenylate cyclase in the anterior pituitary and certain brain regions while a portion of these receptors may be linked to phosphatidylinositol hydrolysis [Kilts, personal communication]. Generally, the magnitude of stimulation of adenylate cyclase by CRF in various brain regions is correlated with the density of CRF receptors. Consistent with the coupling of CRF receptors to adenylate cyclase was the finding that the binding was increased by divalent cations and decreased by guanyl nucleotides [56, 168].

As alluded to above, after binding to its receptor CRF produces rises in intracellular cAMP concentrations. Structure-activity studies with CRF in the anterior pituitary have revealed that the CRF-induced increase in cAMP concentrations is mediated by the carboxy-terminal 27 amino acid sequence [4]; the ED_{50} for the CRF-induced increase in cAMP is 1.3 nM. In cultured rat anterior pituicytes there is a 4-6 fold increase in cAMP concentrations 3 minutes after the addition of CRF, with a maximum 10-15 fold increase over basal concentrations within 30 minutes. The CRF-induced ACTH release from AtT-20 cells is apparently associated with cAMP accumulation. Only a small fraction of total cytosolic cAMP-dependent kinase is required for maximal ACTH secretion. Inhibition of cAMP-dependent kinases with protein kinase inhibitor (PKI) decreases ACTH release in response to CRF. The release of ACTH parallels the intracellular accumulation of cAMP. Not only does CRF stimulate secretion of ACTH, but it also increases POMC mRNA synthesis in both anterior pituitary cell cultures and the AtT-20 cell line [136, 191]. A recent report has found that the CRF-induced elevation of cAMP in cultured anterior pituitary cells can be significantly potentiated by stimulators of protein kinase C [44]. As noted above, extrahypothalamic CRF receptors also appear to be coupled to adenylate cyclase [251, 49].

The regional distribution of CRF binding sites does not exactly correspond with the regional distribution of CRF receptor mediated stimulation of adenylate cyclase. Determination of the stoichiometric relationship between receptor number and cAMP production ("CRF activity index") by calculation of cAMP production per CRF receptor has been calculated. Results are expressed as fmoles cAMP produced/minute/fmole CRF receptor. In the CNS, this CRF activity index finds frontoparietal cortex > midbrain > hippocampus > striatum = cerebellum > hypothalamus > spinal cord > olfactory bulb [57].

One research group [14] has reported that in rat anterior pituitary cultures, CRF (10 nM) induces a thirteen fold increase in cAMP production in ten minutes with a plateau between 20-30 minutes. This increase in cAMP was attenuated by dexamethasone or corticosterone pretreatment. In contrast, another group has reported that while dexamethasone attenuates CRF-induced ACTH release, it does not alter CRF-induced cAMP production, suggesting that the effects of dexamethasone must occur distal to the production of cAMP [79]. CRF-stimulated ACTH release is, as expected, calcium-dependent. The calcium antagonist verapamil apparently has no effect on spontaneous or CRF-induced ACTH release suggesting that intracellular and not extracellular calcium is used during the secretion process. However, a second study using nifedipine indicated that extracellular stores of calcium are required for ACTH secretion. The influx of external calcium ions accelerated cAMP accumulation in response to CRF [81, 82, 154]. The calmodulin inhibitors trifluoperazine and W-7 (N-[6-aminohexyl]-5-chloro-naphthalene-1-sulfomide), inhibit CRF-induced ACTH secretion, but do not diminish CRF-induced cAMP accumulation, providing further evidence that cAMP is not the sole second messenger responsible for the effects of CRF on ACTH secretion [153]. The cAMP analog 8-Br-cAMP and phorbol esters, as well as CRF, increased POMC mRNA content [2]. A role for protein carboxymethylase (PCM) has been suggested in exocytotic secretion. Also, phospholipid methylation of phosphatidylethanolamine to phosphatidylcholine using SAM as the methyl donor has been suggested as a possible membrane transduction mechanism for some receptor induced events. Increased ACTH release, increased phospholipid methylation and increased protein carboxymethylation varied directly with the concentrations of CRF in the media. Moreover, dexamethasone inhibited all three events [96, 110].

Desensitization of the CRF stimulated ACTH release can occur with as little as 10 pM CRF pretreatment. This desensitization manifests itself as a decrease in ACTH released in response to CRF. Interestingly this desensitization can be enhanced by concurrent AVP administration. The desensitization appears to occur at the level of the receptor itself and not distal to it [190, 102]. Ceda and Hoffman [39] then went on to show that with concentrations of dexamethasone greater than 10^{-8} M, no desensitization of CRF-induced ACTH release from cultured rat anterior pituitary cells is observed. This suggests that high ambient plasma glucocorticoid concentrations may explain why the pituitary does not readily desensitize in vivo.

Endocrine Role for CRF

Human fetal hypothalamic extracts contain CRF-like immunoreactivity at 12-13 weeks of gestational age. The content of CRF-like immunoreactivity, however, did not change with increasing gestational age [1]. The ontogeny of CRF responsiveness has been studied. The responsiveness of the anterior pituitary to exogenous CRF first appears at 20 weeks of gestation in humans. However, CRF has no effect on β-endorphin or α-MSH release from the neurointermediate lobe at any time during gestation [74]. In the sheep, IV CRF increases plasma ACTH and cortisol concentrations in the fetus up to 23 days prior to birth [140]. There is an increased sensitivity to CRF at parturition [90, 140]. CRF-containing neurons were detected by immunohistochemistry in the fetal rat paraventricular nucleus after 18 days of gestation. Immediately after birth, the pituitary secretes ACTH, contains numbers of CRF receptors similar to the adult, and responds to CRF both in vivo and <u>in vitro</u>, though with a somewhat diminished sensitivity to the peptide when compared to adults. Recent evidence suggests that the CRF system undergoes a transitory regression postnatally comparable to that of the adrenal cortex. This is followed by an accumulation of CRF in hypothalamic fibers and perikarya [36, 213].

Numerous studies have shown that glucocorticoids can abolish both CRF and ACTH secretion. The mechanism(s) of this negative feedback are multiple and complex. The latency period of glucocorticoid mediated negative feedback occurs within minutes at the level of the anterior pituitary (ACTH secretion), but there is a longer latency period at both the level of the hypothalamus and POMC transcription in the pituitary [71, 266, 194, 212]. The fast feedback does not seem to be mediated through the activation of inhibitory neural pathways. It may result from an alteration of calcium flux that may stabilize the cell membrane to inhibit ACTH release in the presence of glucocorticoids. Delayed feedback may represent inhibition of both ACTH synthesis and release [114]. Plasma corticosterone concentrations of 8-12 µg/dl suppress the increase in portal plasma CRF concentrations induced by nitroprusside, a hypotensive agent. Only at corticosterone concentrations of 40 µg/dl were basal portal plasma concentrations of CRF reduced [182].

It has been suggested that CRF may modulate its own release via retrograde flow in the portal vessels, acting as an ultrashort negative feedback modulator on CRF terminals. However, two reports from McCann's group [163, 164] have not found any evidence for an ultrashort negative feedback loop. Intraventricular oCRF in doses too low to elevate plasma ACTH directly did not decrease plasma ACTH concentrations prior to ether stress. These animals did, however, show an enhanced response to ether stress compared to controls suggesting that a positive ultrashort feedback loop may be activated during stress.

There is little doubt that CRF is the major physiological regulator of ACTH secretion. The concentration of CRF in the portal blood of pentobarbital-anesthetized rats, using an antisera generated against oCRF, was approximately 100 pM; using an anti-rCRF antibody the values were roughly equivalent [73]. Plotsky found that hemorrhage (15% of estimated blood volume) induced a two-fold rise in the concentration of CRF in hypophyseal portal plasma. This rise was abolished by dexamethasone pretreatment. The basal secretory rate was 1.61 ± 0.7 pg/minute and this was not altered by dexamethasone pretreatment [177]. Both intravenous and intracerebroventricular (ICV) CRF injections stimulate the release of ACTH and β-endorphin from the adenohypophysis; these effects are abolished by dexamethasone pretreatment [58, 207, 38]. In addition, CRF has been shown to increase the rate of synthesis of ACTH, as determined by increases in POMC mRNA in pituitary corticotrophs. CRF has also been shown to possess trophic effects as well. Long-term CRF administration is capable of increasing the number of pituitary corticotrophs as well as increases in POMC mRNA [72]. The effects of CRF on ACTH release can be potentiated by a number of weaker ACTH secretagogues including vasopressin, oxytocin, epinephrine, norepinephrine and angiotensin II [257, 139]. These effects can be blocked by immunoneutralization of CRF with intravenously administered CRF antisera [193]. The potency of ovine CRF and rat/human CRF in releasing ACTH are comparable, but the duration of action of oCRF is somewhat longer [271]. Cells from the AtT-20/D16-16 mouse pituitary tumor cell line are also responsive to

CRF stimulation in a manner similar to primary cultures of anterior pituitary cells [109]. These AtT-20 cells have served as a useful model system for studying the biochemistry of CRF mediated events involved in ACTH release and synthesis.

There is some evidence that CRF increases corticosterone secretion in rats not only by stimulating ACTH secretion, but also by increasing adrenocortical responsiveness to ACTH [53], though pharmacological doses of CRF were required. However, Rivier et al. [194] were unable to demonstrate the same effect.

Ovine CRF (8 μg/kg IV) in pentobarbital anesthetized rats not only increased plasma ACTH and corticosterone concentrations, but also those of plasma aldosterone and 18-hydroxycorticosterone [142]. Although, oCRF has been reported to release α-MSH in rats in vivo, this effect was not blocked by dexamethasone [186]. Another report utilizing frog neurointermediate lobe indicated that oCRF had no effect on α-MSH release [250].

The ICV administration of CRF in the rat produces a dose-dependent decrease in LH, but not FSH, secretion presumably via a CNS mechanism. Nikolarakis [160] has recently shown a dose-dependent suppression of basal LH-RH release in response to CRF in rat hypothalamic slices in vitro. When administered IV, CRF does not alter FSH plasma concentrations in the rat or human. It is unclear as to whether IV CRF decreases or has no effect on plasma LH concentrations [198, 202, 162]. Chronic exposure to IV CRF decreased testosterone concentrations and seminal vesicle weights. This effect was not seen in adrenalectomized animals suggesting that, increases in circulating concentrations of adrenal steroids following CRF may in part be responsible for the CRF-induced inhibition of sexual behavior [205].

Conflicting results exist concerning the effects of CRF on growth hormone (GH) secretion. Centrally administered CRF has been reported to decrease GH release, possibly by increasing somatostatin release. Schulte reported that IV CRF increased plasma GH concentrations in non-human primates [199, 222, 203, 120]. In man, IV CRF in general produces no effect on GH secretion [100, 83].

Ovine CRF has been reported to stimulate secretion of somatostatin from dispersed cells of fetal brain, and from median eminence fragments in vitro [3, 169]. Somatostatin itself has been reported to block CRF-induced release of POMC-derived peptides from the rat neurointermediate lobe but not from the anterior pituitary [128]. In contrast, Litvin et al. [137] reported that somatostatin decreases CRF-induced ACTH release from the anterior pituitary. This occurs presumably by inhibiting adenylate cyclase thereby preventing cAMP-dependent protein kinases from phosphorylating proteins. However, under conditions where the activity of cAMP dependent kinases are sufficient to induce ACTH release, high concentrations of somatostatin can inhibit ACTH secretion by an independent mechanism.

Recently [161], CRF has been shown to stimulate β-endorphin and dynorphin release from rat hypothalamic slices.

Numerous investigators have demonstrated that arginine-vasopressin (AVP) potentiates the effect of CRF on ACTH release. Thus the combination of CRF and AVP produce greater plasma ACTH elevations than the sum of either peptide alone. The potency of vasopressin analogs to enhance the action of CRF is not related to their reported vasopressor or antidiuretic activity. This provides some evidence that the structural requirements for potentiation of CRF action may differ from the action of AVP at other receptor sites. In contrast, others have reported that the CRF activity of AVP is clearly related to its pressor activity [123, 152, 45, 68, 189, 196, 86, 138, 185].

There is no doubt that separate receptors mediate the action of AVP and CRF on ACTH release. Giguere suggested that the potentiation of CRF-induced ACTH release by AVP probably occurs, at least in part, through potentiation of intracellular cAMP accumulation, but AVP alone does not alter cAMP levels [80]. However, Holmes [105] found that vasopressin does not alter CRF-stimulated adenylate cyclase activity. Two different receptors have been described that mediate the peripheral action of AVP. The V_1 receptor mediates the pressor activity of the peptide; the V_2 receptor, apparently mediates its antidiuretic effect. Whereas Rivier has evidence that the V_1 receptor subtype may mediate the peptide's action on corticotrophs, a Hungarian group reported that neither the classical V_1 or V_2 receptor is responsible for its CRF potentiating effect [204, 200, 9].

The ratio of AVP:CRF release from the median eminence in vitro increases from 2:1 in sham-operated rats to 8:1 in adrenalectomized rats [106]. This suggests that AVP may be the predominant corticotropic stimulus in adrenalectomized rats. However, administration of antisera to oCRF or rat/human CRF suppressed the elevations in ACTH following adrenalectomy in rats, whereas antibodies to AVP or AVP antagonists had no effect. This indicates that CRF plays the major role in adrenalectomy-induced ACTH secretion [92]. Plotsky et al. [181] measured the concentrations of CRF and AVP in hypophyseal portal blood in response to insulin-induced hypoglycemia. Their results suggest that CRF functions in a permissive role allowing expression of the weaker ACTH-releasing activity of AVP and other secretagogues. Portal concentrations of AVP and OT were not altered following nitroprusside-induced hypotension. This suggests that CRF plays the major role in the elevation of plasma ACTH in this paradigm [182]. Immunoneutralization of AVP, by ICV injection of AVP antisera, resulted in a large increase in the concentration of CRF in the portal vessel system. This led Plotsky and his colleagues to postulate that endogenous AVP may be inhibitory at the hypothalamic level of the HPA axis, while it is stimulatory at the level of the anterior pituitary [180].

Although oxytocin (OT) has been reported to slightly increase basal ACTH secretion, like AVP, it also potentiates the ACTH response to CRF [76]. Immunoneutralization of OT has been reported to result in a 59% decrease in ACTH secretion in response to stress [77]. There is also evidence that epinephrine, by increasing cAMP production in response to CRF, potentiates the effect of the releasing factor on ACTH release; this effect appears to be mediated by an α-adrenergic mechanism in vitro [82]. Immunoneutralization of CRF abolishes these effects of both OT and epinephrine suggesting that these agents somehow interact directly with endogenous CRF [202]. As is the case with AVP, there is also evidence that CNS epinephrine inhibits HPA activity. Recently epinephrine-containing nerve terminals have been shown to innervate CRF-containing neurons in the PVN [135].

When administered directly into the CNS, CRF produces effects that are apparently not mediated by activation of the HPA axis. Thus, ICV CRF (19 nmoles) produces physiological changes not unlike those observed in response to stress. These include: increases in heart rate, mean arterial pressure (MAP), oxygen consumption, blood glucose

and plasma catecholamines, all mediated by an increase in central
sympathetic outflow [22, 23, 24, 69]. Microinjection studies suggest
that no single brain area is responsible for these responses to
exogenous CRF administration [27]. In a recent report, the increases
in heart rate, MAP and locomotion following ICV CRF administration were
blocked by pretreatment with IV naloxone. This is the first time
naloxone has been reported to block the effects of CRF; this suggests
that the increased sympathetic activation is under opioid control
[215]. In the Rhesus monkey however, Insel et al. [112] did not
observe any change in heart rate, mean arterial pressure or plasma
norepinephrine concentrations following ICV CRF in doses as high as 60
µg/kg. Valentino et al. [259] reported that while both HPA and LC
activity were increased following ICV CRF (3 µg), there were no
concomitant changes in blood pressure. This observation demonstrates
that an increase in spontaneous LC activity does not necessarily result
in an increase in blood pressure.

IV CRF produces a slight decrease in mean arterial pressure, probably
due to increased mesenteric blood flow, and a slight increase in heart
rate [24, 118, 252] but this effect requires pharmacological doses of
the peptide.

In a recent report, Bueno [35] found that ICV, but not IV, CRF
(20-100 ng/kg) suppressed gastrointestinal motor activity, an effect
also observed when animals are exposed to stress. Intracisternal
administration of CRF acts within the brain to inhibit gastric acid
secretion through vagal and adrenal mechanisms, not mediated by
activation of the HPA axis [247].

Recent evidence has suggested that there is a link between the
neuroendocrine and immune systems and these findings have been reviewed
[89]. Blalock et al. [267] reported that both hepatocyte-stimulating
factor and interleukin-I (IL-1) stimulated the release of ACTH from
AtT-20 pituitary cells. The latter agent was equipotent with the
combination of CRF and AVP in its ability to stimulate ACTH release.
Another research group has reported that IL-1 increases plasma concentrations of ACTH and corticosterone in vivo [13]. Blalock and his
colleagues also reported that leukocytes can produce and secrete ACTH
and β-endorphin in response to CRF [232]. However, neither our group
[192] nor DeSouza [personal communication] have been able to identify
CRF receptors on lymphocytes.

CRF and Stress

Stress-induced increases in plasma ACTH concentrations are due to
release of several neuroregulators including CRF, AVP, OT, angiotensin
II, VIP, PHI, epinephrine and norepinephrine. However, the evidence
for CRF playing the predominant role is provided by the finding that
this stress-induced release of ACTH can almost completely be blocked by
CRF antiserum and/or a CRF antagonist (α-helical oCRF$_{9-41}$). Both in
vivo and in vitro, epinephrine-stimulated release of ACTH is thought to
be mediated by a β-adrenergic mechanism [249, 132, 195, 157]. This is
in contrast to the work of Giguere [82] mentioned earlier. Central
administration of the CRF antagonist reverses the stress-induced
inhibition of LH and GH release and the rise in plasma epinephrine
concentrations [203, 206, 26], suggesting that CRF also mediates these
stress responses.

Pituitary cell suspensions obtained from acutely stressed animals exhibit a blunted ACTH and β-endorphin (0.01 mM) response to CRF in vitro. This could be due at least in part, to high circulating glucocorticoids at the time of sacrifice. Pituitary cell suspensions from chronically stressed (14 days of footshock) exhibited no change in sensitivity to CRF and do not exhibit a blunted ACTH response to CRF even when acutely stressed just prior to sacrifice. In fact, these animals tended to exhibit a potentiation of ACTH and β-endorphin release into the media in vitro. The failure of an acute stressor to alter the ACTH response to CRF may indicate a down regulation of steroid feedback on the pituitary [272] or down regulation of the CRF receptors on the corticotrophs. It is evident that during chronic stress, complex adaptive mechanisms are probably at work in the anterior pituitary, CNS and adrenal.

Recently we [40] have scrutinized, in detail, alterations in the concentrations of CRF in 36 different micropunched rat brain regions following exposure to either a single acute (3 hour immobilization at 4°C) or chronic unpredictable stressors (14 days). The results with CRF are summarized in Table 2 and Figure 2.

Acute stress decreased the concentration of CRF in the arcuate nucleus/median eminence (ARC/ME) and medial preoptic (MPO) nucleus; in contrast the concentration of CRF in the LC was markedly increased. Chronically stressed (daily unpredictable stressors) rats exhibited similar changes in CRF content in the ARC/ME, and the LC and, in addition, exhibited an increase in CRF concentration in the anterior hypothalamic and periventricular nuclei. A significant decrease in CRF concentration was found in the dorsal vagal complex of the chronically stressed animals. Although not statistically significant, there was a trend for an increase in CRF concentration in the bed nucleus of the stria terminalis after both acute and chronic stress. It appears that the rate of synthesis of CRF in neurons that project to the ME is unable to keep up with its release during chronic stress because CRF-LI in the ARC/ME remained appreciably diminished when compared to the controls. The increases of CRF-LI in the LC are more difficult to explain. Measurement of CRF concentrations alone cannot distinguish between alterations in CRF synthesis, release or degradation. However, the fact that the LC was one of the few regions to show stress-induced alterations is intriguing in light of the evidence showing that CRF alters LC neuronal firing rates, and may be involved in modulating the LC noradrenergic neurons during stress.

Behavioral Effects of Centrally Administered CRF

CRF administered centrally produces a variety of behavioral effects that have conclusively been shown not to be mediated by stimulation of the pituitary-adrenal axis. These behaviors are generally insensitive to dexamethasone administration [17, 19] and are not abolished by hypophysectomy. This area is comprehensively described in this volume by Thatcher-Britton and Koob; we therefore briefly review the findings relevant to affective disorders here.

When administered ICV in low doses, CRF increases locomotor activity. The effects of CRF on locomotion are similar to those of mild stress. This locomotor activation is not altered by opiates or the opiate receptor antagonist naloxone. Dopamine receptor antagonists block the CRF-induced locomotor activity only at cateleptic doses [124, 59, 245, 126, 243]. Recently, Kalivas [119] has found that increases

Table 2. Effect of acute and chronic stress on adrenal weight, plasma ACTH and corticosterone concentration, and pituitary ACTH content

	Controls	Acute stress	Chronic stress
Adrenal weight (mg ± SEM)	42 ± 2	43 ± 2	51 ± 2*
Plasma ACTH (pg/ml ± SEM)	123 ± 9	186 ± 21**	122 ± 6
Plasma corticosterone (µg/dl ± SEM)	16 ± 3	51 ± 5***	29 ± 5*
Pituitary ACTH content (ng/pituitary ± SEM)	4.03 ± 0.41	3.28 ± 0.30	3.40 ± 0.34

Data were analyzed by 1-way ANOVA followed by Scheffe's test for intergroup differences. Each group consisted of 10 subjects.

*Significantly different from controls and acute stress group, $p < 0.05$.
**Significantly different from controls and chronic stress group, $p < 0.05$.
***Significantly different from controls and chronic stress group, $p < 0.01$.

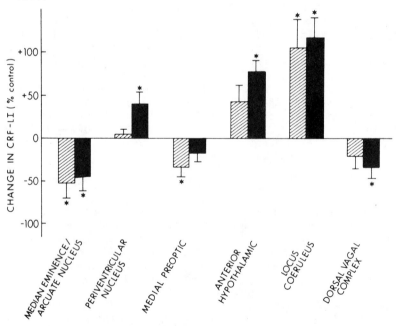

Figure 2. Percentage from baseline of stress-induced change in CRF-LI concentration. Hatched bars represent acute stress. Solid bars represent chronic stress. *, Significantly different from controls, $p < 0.05$.

in locomotor behavior following direct injection of CRF (.01-0.1 nmoles) into the ventral tegmental area of the rat are not blocked by pretreatment with the dopamine receptor antagonist haloperidol. He also found a decrease in dopamine metabolism in the prefrontal cortex, an effect opposite to that of stress, but not in the striatum or nucleus accumbens. This further confirms Koob's finding that the loco-motor activating effects of CRF are not mediated by the mesolimbic and mesocortical dopamine systems. This also suggests that the "stress-like" effects of CRF are neurochemically different from those produced by other stressors (e.g., restraint, shock, etc.). Another finding that suggests that the behavioral effects of CRF are neurochemically distinct is the observation that, although ICV-CRF produces certain stress-like behaviors, there is no evidence that it produces analgesia which is well known to occur after stress [226]. Several investigators have noted the similarities in the behavioral effects of centrally administered CRF and a variety of stress-associated behaviors; CRF may act at least in part through activation of central catecholaminergic systems [Dunn (personal communication), 16].

Infusion of CRF into the arcuate-ventromedial area of the mediobasal hypothalamus and the mesencephalic grey area potently suppresses sexual behavior in the female rat. Microinjection into the medial preoptic area (MPOA), also inhibited lordosis behavior. CRF immunoneutraliza-tion increased lordosis behavior, which was blocked by an LH-RH antagonist. This suggests that the effects of CRF on sexual behavior may be mediated at neurons that have receptors for both LH-RH and CRF in the hypothalamus by inhibiting LH-RH release. These may be the LH-RH containing neurons themselves [229, 230].

CRF decreases food consumption induced by food deprivation as well as food consumption induced by a variety of drugs including muscimol, norepinephrine, dynorphin 1-13, ethylketoclyclazocine, and insulin [131, 148, 85, 210].

As Koob has emphasized, ICV CRF produces behavioral alterations consistent with increased "emotionality". These alterations include: increased locomotion, sniffing, grooming and rearing, all of which are consistent with behavioral arousal. CRF potentiates the effects of exposure to a novel environment. These "anxiogenic" effects of CRF are opposite to those of anxiolytics and are reversed with low doses of chlordiazepoxide. Thus CRF appears to increase emotionality [125, 126, 127, 243, 118, 262]. Consistent with the anxiogenic properties of this peptide is the recent observation that CRF potentiates the acoustic startle response, an effect also blocked by chlordiazepoxide [246]. Chlordiazepoxide and ethanol both produced a dose-dependent reversal of CRF-induced response suppression in the conflict model of anxiety [18, 21]. The CRF antagonist, α-helical CRF$_{9-41}$, also attenuated the effects of CRF in the conflict test without producing any overt behavioral effects of its own [20].

Because CRF has clear activating or "arousal" properties, it might enhance the ability of an animal to acquire a learned response. In a familiar environment, CRF administered prior to the daily acquisition of an appetively motivated visual discrimination task significantly improved acquisition [127].

Release

As noted earlier, CRF fulfills many of the requisite neurotransmitter

criteria. Calcium-dependent release from nerve terminals in response
to physiological depolarizing agents is generally accepted as another
necessary criterion for a substance to be considered a neurotransmitter. Using a sensitive and specific RIA, we demonstrated CRF
release in response to depolarizing concentrations of potassium. This
phenomenon was observed not only in hypothalamus, but also in amygdala,
midbrain and striatum as well [233]. These results are illustrated in
Figures 3 and 4.

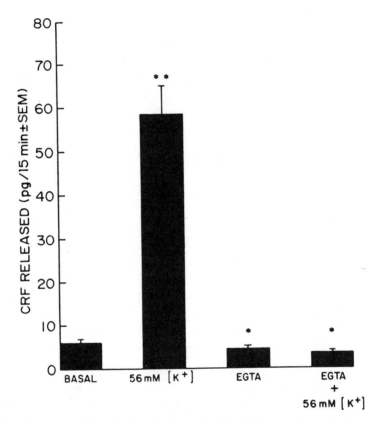

Figure 3. Calcium-dependent release of CRF-LI from the rat
hypothalamus in vitro. CRF release into the medium was measured by RIA
during a 15-min incubation at 37°C and is expressed as the average ±
SEM of triplicate determinations from four separate experiments. CRF
is expressed as picograms released from a single hypothalamus per tube
during a 15-min incubation (average weight of hypothalamus, 50 ± 3 mg).
*, P < 0.05; **, P < 0.01 (vs. basal release).

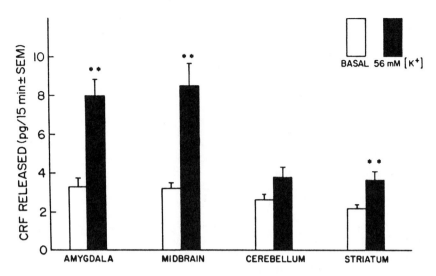

Figure 4. Potassium-evoked release of CRF-like immunoreactivity from various brain regions in vitro. CRF release in response to 56 mM K$^+$ was determined during a 15-min incubation and is expressed as the average ± SEM of triplicate determinations from three separate experiments. CRF is expressed as picograms released from the brain region of a single rat, although usually tissue from two rats was used per tube. **, P < 0.01 vs. basal release.

Considerable controversy currently exists concerning the role of various neurotransmitters in regulating secretion of hypothalamic CRF.

Utilizing immunocytochemical methods, Liposits has demonstrated tyrosine hydroxylase immunoreactive nerve terminals (a marker of catecholamine neurons) innervating CRF-containing perikarya in the PVN. He has also found phenethylamine-N-methyl transferase (PNMT) immunoreactive nerve terminals, a marker of epinephrine-containing neurons, that arise from the C_1 (ventral lateral medulla) and C_2 (dorsal vagal complex) cell groups, establishing synaptic contact with PVN CRF perikarya [134, 135]. These findings provide the anatomical evidence for direct dopaminergic, noradrenergic and/or adrenergic control of CRF release.

The pertinent literature concerning regulation of CRF release from in vivo and in vitro studies are summarized in Tables 3 and 4, and the many discrepancies are clear. The majority of these studies were conducted prior to identification of CRF and utilized bioassay methods to measure CRF release. Although bioassays can be quite sensitive, they lack specificity; various secretagogues other than CRF itself possess CRF-like activity, e.g. vasopressin, oxytocin and epinephrine. For this reason, more definitive investigations utilizing specific and sensitive radioimmunoassay methods are now being used to elucidate the control of hypothalamic CRF release. Using a hypothalamic block preparation modeled after the work of Jones, Buckingham and their colleagues, we have demonstrated that both muscarinic and serotonergic agonists stimulate CRF release in vitro. In preliminary studies we have demonstrated that the benzodiazepine alprazolam, an effective anxiolytic and anti-panic agent, attenuates CRF release in response to serotonin. This suggests that alprazolam and other benzodiazepines may reduce HPA axis activity by inhibiting CRF release. This finding has been confirmed by Gold and his colleagues [personal communication].

Electrophysiology

In several studies CRF has been shown to exert predominantly excitatory actions in a variety of brain areas including: the LC [258], hippocampus, cerebral cortex and parts of the hypothalamus. Intracellular recordings from hippocampal slices demonstrated that CRF induced excitation may arise from a reduction of the afterhyperpolarizations (AHP's) following bursts of spikes. Recordings in the presence of TTX indicated that CRF is acting either at the level of the Ca^{++}-dependent, K^+ conductance itself, or at the linkage between this conductance and Ca^{++} influx or Ca^{++} recognition sites [228, 6]. Studies utilizing verapamil (a calcium channel antagonist) would seem to indicate that CRF acts by a transmembrane signalling system to block this Ca^{++}-dependent K^+ conductance. The net result would be a change in the membrane potential closer to depolarization, thereby increasing the likelihood of discharge activity. In contrast to these findings, CRF exerts predominantly inhibitory actions on neurons in the thalamus, lateral septum and PVN of the hypothalamus. In general, neurons excited by iontophoretically applied CRF are inhibited by dopamine and morphine, while those that were inhibited by CRF are excited by these agents [60].

The responses of LC neurons to electrical stimulation of the sciatic nerve usually consists of a brief period of activation followed by an epoch of relative inhibition. ICV CRF attenuated both components of this response demonstrating that the phasic response to noxious stimuli were attenuated with respect to tonic background activity. This attenuation was not linearly related to the CRF-induced increase in spontaneous discharge rate. Of particular interest is the finding that these responses are similar to those observed after ethanol administration, suggesting that ethanol may exert its effects on LC activity by release of CRF [260]. Although these effects are not easily interpreted, they suggest that when the LC is active, the magnitude of responses due to discrete stimuli are decreased in the presence of CRF. Behaviorally, this might manifest itself by an attenuation of LC activity to further discrete stimuli in an already aroused animal. This may be of survival value in animals during periods of arousal or in very stressful situations.

Low doses of centrally administered CRF produce EEG changes suggestive of increased arousal. Higher doses lead to EEG and behavioral signs of seizure activity indistinguishable from those that occur following electrical "kindling" of the amygdala [61]. Weiss and her colleagues [263] found that high doses of ICV CRF (100 µg/day x 5 days) produced major motor seizures in all animals after a delay of 1-5 hours on days 1 and 2. By day five, however, no rats exhibited seizures, suggesting the development of tolerance. After CRF treatment, rats developed amygdala-kindled seizures following electrical stimulation twice as rapidly as vehicle-injected controls. Interestingly, electrically kindled rats were significantly less sensitive to CRF-induced seizures. These findings suggest that CRF-induced seizures are not entirely parallel to amygdala-kindled seizures.

Table 3. Effects of Neurotransmitters, Hormones and Drugs on CRF Release _in vitro_. Numbers refer to citations in bibliography.

	Stimulates CRF Release (+)	Inhibits CRF Release (-)	No Effect on CRF Release (0)
ACETYLCHOLINE	[29, 33, 159, 15, 116]		[62]
nicotinic agonists	[101, 30]		
muscarinic agonists	[101, 30, 241]		
SEROTONERGIC agonists	[33, 29, 30, 115, 116, 104, 156]		[62, 248]
NOREPINEPHRINE	[62]	[62, 29, 241]	[248, 101]
DOPAMINE	[62]		[29, 101]
EPINEPHRINE			[29]
ANGIOTENSIN II	[29, 238, 236]		
MORPHINE	[31, 33]		
β-ENDORPHIN	[33]	[33, 270]	
met-ENKEPHALIN	[31, 33]	[270]	
leu-ENKEPHALIN	[31, 33]	[270]	
DYNORPHIN		[270]	
HISTAMINE			[29, 62, 101]
GABA		[115]	[29, 62, 241]
ACTH 1-39		[240]	
CORTICOSTERONE		[32]	[29]
DEXAMETHASONE		[238]	
ALDOSTERONE		[32]	
ESTROGENS	[32]		
cAMP	[238]		
GLYCINE		[29]	
GLUTAMATE			[29]

Table 4. Effects of Neurotransmitters, Hormones and Drugs on CRF Release _in vivo_. Numbers refer to citations in bibliography.

	Stimulates CRF Release (+)	Inhibits CRF Release (-)	No Effect on CRF Release (0)
ACETYLCHOLINE	[121]		
nicotinic agonists	[121]		
muscarinic agonists	[95]	[121]	
SEROTONIN	[75, 91, 150, 64]		
NOREPINEPHRINE	[234, 78, 10, 63, 65]	[65]	
DOPAMINE		[253, 155]	
EPINEPHRINE	[249]	[261, 208, 145]	
OPIATES sigma	[167]		
mu (morphine sufate)	[242, 94, 34, 173]		
β-endorphin		[183]	
kappa agonists	[94, 173, 113]		
dynorphin		[183]	
met-enkephalin		[188]	
naltrexone	[183]		
HISTAMINE			[37, 225]
ETHANOL	[201]		
GABA		[141, 254]	
VASOPRESSIN		[178]	
SRIF		[25]	
CRF			[179]
ANGIOTENSIN II	[236]		

Clinical Studies with CRF

We shall only briefly touch upon studies of the CRF stimulation test here because they are described in detail elsewhere in this volume in the chapters by Gold and by Holsboer. In human subjects, oCRF is more potent than rat/human CRF because of its longer plasma half-life. There is a dose response relationship for both peptides on plasma ACTH and cortisol concentrations.

While most human studies have shown no serious side effects to intravenously administered CRF, there have been reports of hypotension in normal subjects and serious hypotensive reactions in four individuals with a hypothalamic-pituitary-adrenal dysfunction of one sort or another [98, 99]. This may be due to impurities in certain of the commercially available CRF preparations.

Measurement of plasma CRF-like immunoreactivity has recently been accomplished using immunoaffinity chromatography. Suda has reported basal plasma concentrations in normal subjects of 6 ± 0.5 pg/ml (mean $\pm$ SD). Plasma CRF concentrations were reportedly altered by stress, negative feedback and circadian rhythms. As expected, plasma CRF concentrations were increased in Addison's disease (due to the lack of glucocorticoid negative feedback) and very low but detectable (1-3 pg/ml) concentrations were found in patients with Cushing's syndrome, as well as in patients treated with glucocorticoids. These data suggest that a major component of the plasma CRF-LI is of hypothalamic origin [239]. However, Charlton et al. [41] were unable to find any diurnal variations in plasma CRF concentrations nor any correlations between plasma cortisol and CRF concentrations.

Of pertinence to this chapter is the finding by Widerlov [265] that the plasma from 10 drug-free depressed patients was found to contain significantly elevated concentrations of CRF when compared to normal controls. However, this is discordant with the results of Charlton et al. [41]. Schulte [223] found that continuous IV administration of CRF to human volunteers for 8-24 hours increases ACTH and plasma cortisol concentrations in a pattern similar to that observed in depressed patients. Despite the constant levels of plasma CRF obtained during the infusion, a persistent circadian rhythm of ACTH was observed. Thus, the circadian variation of HPA axis activity cannot adequately be explained by circadian periodicity of endogenous CRF release alone.

Cushing's syndrome can be divided into three types: that due to pituitary hypersecretion of ACTH (Cushing's disease); hypersecretion secondary to ectopic ACTH or CRF secretion; and hypercortisolism from autonomous secretion of cortisol by the adrenal gland. The differential diagnosis between the two types of ACTH dependent Cushing's syndrome is often difficult. The CRF stimulation test appears to differentiate between the three forms of Cushing's syndrome. Patients with pituitary Cushing's disease respond to IV CRF with normal or increased plasma ACTH and cortisol concentrations despite high circulating levels of cortisol. Patients with ectopic ACTH syndrome usually fail to respond to exogenous CRF. As noted, the CRF stimulation test has been studied in patients with psychiatric disorders. As a group, patients with major depression exhibit a blunted ACTH response to CRF when compared to normal controls [83, 84, 107, 108]. This suggests either that the negative feedback system is intact and that the high circulating concentrations of cortisol are responsible for the blunted ACTH response, or alternatively, the blunted ACTH response is due to

desensitization of pituitary CRF receptors. In any case, the
hypercortisolism seen in this subgroup may well be due to chronic CRF
hypersecretion [151, 176, 221, 12, 83, 84, 107, 108, 42]. A blunted
ACTH response to CRF is also observed in patients with anorexia nervosa
[111, 84].

We attempted, in two studies, to directly test the hypothesis that
CRF is hypersecreted in depressed patients by measuring the concentrations of the peptide in CSF of drug-free patients and controls. In
our first study (Figure 5), eleven of 23 depressed patients had higher
CSF CRF values than the highest normal controls. In contrast, there
was no difference in CSF CRF concentrations in schizophrenic patients
or patients with dementia when compared with normal controls [158]. We
have now confirmed this finding in a second study of 54 depressed
patients and 138 controls (Figure 6); CSF CRF concentrations were
markedly elevated (almost twofold) in the depressed patients when compared to both controls and nondepressed psychiatric patients [11]. The
non-normal distribution of CSF CRF values suggests that there may be a
subgroup of depressed patients with elevated CSF CRF values. In both
of these studies, elevated CSF CRF values were not correlated with
dexamethasone nonsuppressors; however, Gold and his colleagues have
recently found a significant correlation between post-dexamethasone
plasma cortisol and CSF CRF concentrations [Roy et al., in press].

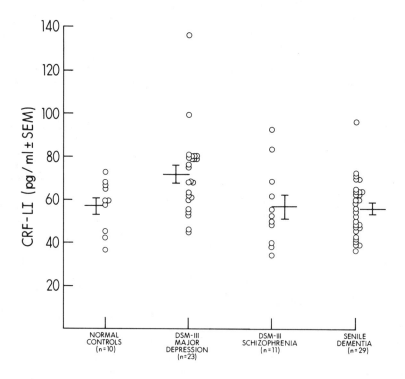

Figure 5. Concentration of CRF-LI in CSF of normal controls (5 males
and 5 females), DSM-III major depression (13 males and 10 females),
DSM-III schizophrenia (8 females and 3 males), and senile dementia
(DSM-III primary degenerative dementia or multi-infarct dementia, or

both, 20 females and 9 males). Because the data distribution in the depressed patients was slightly skewed, the data were analyzed by both parametric (ANOVA and Student-Newman-Keuls test) and nonparametric (Mann-Whitney U test) methods. By both methods of CSF CRF-LI concentrations were significantly elevated in the depressed patients when compared to the other diagnostic groups and the normal controls (P < 0.05, ANOVA and Student-Newman-Keuls test; P < 0.025, Mann-Whitney U test).

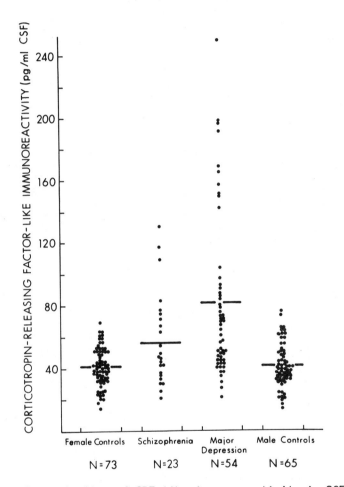

Figure 6. Concentration of CRF-like immunoreactivity in CSF of female neurologic controls (n = 73), patients with DSM-III schizophrenia (n = 27), patients with DSM-III major depression (n = 54) and male neurologic controls (n = 65). Respective group mean concentrations of CRF-LI expressed as picograms per milliliter CSF were 40.64 ± 1.43, 57.77 ± 5.96, 80.66 ± 7.07 and 40.91 ± 1.77. Using ANOVA and Newman-Keuls tests for statistical significance, the mean CSF concentrations of CRF-LI in the patients with major depression were significantly elevated (p < 0.001) compared to controls, while the schizophrenic patients were significantly elevated at the p < 0.05 level when compared to controls. The depressed group was also

significantly elevated (p < 0.01) relative to the schizophrenic group. Amer. J. Psychiatry (in press), the American Psychiatric Association. Reprinted by permission.

The above CSF data, taken together with the plethora of behavioral data from animal studies (vide supra) led us to hypothesize that hypersecretion of CRF would produce a reduction in the number of CRF binding sites (down-regulation, decreased Bmax) in the CNS of depressed individuals. With this in mind, we have measured the number (Bmax) and affinity (K_D) of high affinity CRF binding sites in the frontal cortex of suicide victims, some of whom were certainly depressed, and age- and sex-matched controls. Scatchard analysis revealed no difference between the affinity (K_D) for the radioligand in the two groups. However, a significant decrease (23%, p = 0.020) in CRF receptor density was found in the suicide group. No significant correlations were found between the Bmax for CRF and sex, age or post-mortem delay. These findings are concordant with the hypothesis that CRF is hypersecreted in suicide victims as evidenced by the decrease (down regulation) of CRF binding sites.

The clinical findings reviewed in the last section suggest that CRF systems throughout the brain may be pathologically altered in certain psychiatric disorders, including depression and anorexia nervosa. This hypothesis is rendered plausible by both the clinical studies and the preclinical studies in which centrally administered CRF in animals produced behavioral effects similar to those seen in depressed patients, e.g. decreased food consumption, disturbed sleep patterns, decreased sexual behavior. It is unclear at this time whether a hyperfunctioning CRF system is a result of the postulated alterations in monoaminergic systems in depression or whether changes in monoaminergic circuits are secondary to CRF hypersecretion.

Acknowledgements

The authors are supported by NIMH MH-42088, MH-39415, MH-40524, MH-40159, NIA AG-05128, NIEHS Training Grant ES-07031. CBN is the recipient of a Nanaline H. Duke Scholars award from Duke University Medical Center. We are grateful to Shelia Walker for preparation of this manuscript.

REFERENCES

1. Ackland, J. F., Ratter, S. J., Bourne, G. L., and Rees, L. H. (1986): J. Endocrinol., 108:171-180.
2. Affolter, H.-U., and Reisine, T. (1985): J. Biol. Chem., 260:15477-15481.
3. Aguila, M. C., and McCann, S. M. (1985): Brain Res., 348:180-182.
4. Aguilera, G., Harwood, J. P., Wilson, J. X., Morell, J., Brown, J. H., and Catt, K. J. (1983): J. Biol. Chem., 258:8039-8045.
5. Aguilera, G., Millan, M. A., Hauger, R. L., Harwood, J. P., and Catt, K. J. (1986): Proc. Int. Union Physiol. Sci., Vol. XVI, XXXth Congress.
6. Aldenhoff, J. B., Gruol, D. L., Rivier, J., Vale, W., and Siggins, G.R. (1983): Science, 221:875-877.

7. Alonso, G., Szafarczyk, A., and Assenmacher, I. (1986): Exp. Brain Res., 61:497-505.
8. Antoni, F. A., Palkovits, M., Makara, G. B., Linton, E. A., Lowry, P. J., and Kiss, J. Z. (1983): Neuroendocrinology, 36:415-423.
9. Antoni, F. A., Holmes, M. C., Makara, G. B., Karteszi, M., and Laszlo, F. A. (1984): Peptides, 5:519-522.
10. Bakke, H. K., Murison, R., and Walther, B. (1986): Brain Res., 368:256-261.
11. Banki, C. M., Bissette, G., Arato, M., O'Connor, L., and Nemeroff, C. B. Am. J. Psych., (in press).
12. Belsky, J. L., Cuello, B., Swanson, L. W., Simmons, D. M., Jarrett, R. M., and Braza, F. (1985): J. Clin. Endocrinol. Met., 60:496-500.
13. Besedovsky, H., del Rey, A., Sorkin, E., and Dinarello, C. A., (1986): Science, 233:652-654.
14. Bilezikjian, L. M, and Vale, W. W. (1983): Endocrinology, 113:657-662.
15. Bradbury, M. W. B., Burden, J., Hillhouse, E. W., and Jones, M. T. (1974): J. Physiol., 239:269-283.
16. Britton, D. R., Koob, G. F., Rivier, J., and Vale, W. (1982): Life Sci., 31:363-367.
17. Britton, D. R., Varela, M., Garcia, A., and Rosenthal, M. (1986): Life Sci., 38:211-216.
18. Britton, K. T-., Morgan, J., Rivier, J., Vale, W., and Koob, G. F. (1985): Psychopharmacology, 86:170-174.
19. Britton, K. T-., Lee, G., Dana, R., Risch, S. C., and Koob, G. F. (1986): Life Sci., 39:1281-1286.
20. Britton, K. T-., Lee, G., Vale, W., Rivier, J., and Koob, G. F. (1986): Brain Res., 369:303-306.
21. Britton, K. T-., and Koob, G. F. (1986): Reg. Peptides, 16:315-320.
22. Brown, M. R., Fisher, L. A., Rivier, J., Spiess, J., Rivier, C., and Vale, W. (1982): Life Sci., 30:207-210.
23. Brown, M. R., Fisher, L. A., Spiess, J., Rivier, C., Rivier, J., and Vale, W. (1982): Endocrinology, 111:928-931.
24. Brown, M. R., and Fisher, L. A. (1983): Brain Res., 280:75-79.
25. Brown, M. R., Rivier, C., and Vale, W. (1984): Endocrinology, 114:1546-1549.
26. Brown, M. R., Fisher, L. A., Webb, V., Vale, W. W., and Rivier, J. E. (1985): Brain Res., 328:355-357.
27. Brown, M. (1986): Brain Res., 399:10-14.
28. Bruhn, T. O., Engeland, W. C., Anthony, E. L. P., Gann, D. S., and Jackson, I. M. D. (1987): Endocrinology, 120:25-33.
29. Buckingham, J. C., and Hodges, J. R. (1977): J. Physiol., 272:469-479.
30. Buckingham, J. C., and Hodges, J. R. (1979): J. Physiol., 290:421-431.
31. Buckingham, J. C. (1982): Neuroendocrinology, 35:111-116.
32. Buckingham, J. C. (1982): J. Endocrinol., 93:123-132.
33. Buckingham, J. C. (1986): Neuroendocrinology, 42:148-152.
34. Buckingham, J. C., and Cooper, T. A. (1986): Neuroendocrinology, 42:421-426.
35. Bueno, L., and Fioramonti, J. (1986): Peptides, 7:73-77.

36. Bugnon, C., Fellmann, D., Gouget, A., and Cardot, J. (1982):
    Nature, 298:159-161.
37. Cacabelos, R., Yamatodani, A., Fukui, H., Watanabe, T.,
    Hariguchi, S., Nishimura, T., and Wada, H. (1985): Biogenic
    Amines, 3:9-19.
38. Carsia, R. V., Weber, H., and Perez, F. M., Jr. (1986):
    Endocrinology, 118:143-148.
39. Ceda, G. P., and Hoffman, A. R. (1986): Endocrinology,
    118:58-62.
40. Chappell, P. B., Smith, M. A., Kilts, C. D., Bissette, G.,
    Ritchie, J., Anderson, C., and Nemeroff, C. B. (1986): J.
    Neurosci., 6:2908-2914.
41. Charlton, B. G., Leake, A., Ferrier, I. N., Linton, E. A., and
    Lowry, P. J. (1986): Lancet, 161-162.
42. Chrousos, G. P., Schuermeyer, T. H., Doppman, J., Oldfield, E.
    H., Schulte, H. M., Gold, P. W., and Loriaux, D. L. (1985):
    Ann. Intern. Med., 102:344-358.
43. Crawley, J. N., Olschowka, J. A., Diz, D. I., and Jacobowitz, D.
    M. (1985): Peptides, 6:891-901.
44. Cronin, M. J., Zysk, J. R., and Baertschi, A. J. (1986):
    Peptides, 7:935-938.
45. Culler, M. D., Turkelson, C. M., Thomas, C. R., and Arimura, A.
    (1983): Proc. Soc. Exp. Biol. Med., 173:264-269.
46. Cummings, S., Elde, R., Ells, J., and Lindall, A. (1983): J.
    Neurosci., 3:1355-1368.
47. Daikoku, S., Okamura, Y., Kawano, H., Tsuruo, Y., Maegawa, M.,
    and Shibasaki, T. (1984): Cell Tissue Res., 238:539-544.
48. Daikoku, S., Okamura, Y., Kawano, H., Usuruo, Y., Maegawa, M.,
    and Shibasaki, T. (1985): Cell Tissue Res., 240:575-584.
49. Dave, J. R., Eiden, L. E., and Eskay, R. L. (1985):
    Endocrinology, 116:2152-2159.
50. Dave, J. R., and Eskay, R. L. (1986): Biochem. Biophys. Res.
    Comm., 136:137-144.
51. De Souza, E. B., Perrin, M. H., Insel, T. R., Rivier, J., Vale,
    W. W., and Kuhar, M. J. (1984): Science, 224:1449-1451.
52. De Souza, E. B., Perrin, M. H., Rivier, J., Vale, W. W., and
    Kuhar, M. J. (1984): Brain Res., 296:202-207.
53. De Souza, E., and Van Loon, G. R. (1984): Experientia,
    40:1004-1006.
54. De Souza, E. B., Insel, T. R., Perrin, M. H., Rivier, J., Vale,
    W. W., and Kuhar, M. J. (1985): Neurosci. Lett., 56:121-128.
55. De Souza, E. B., Insel, T. R., Perrin, M. H., Rivier, J., Vale,
    W. W., and Kuhar, M. J. (1985): J. Neurosci., 5:3189-3203.
56. De Souza, E. B. (1987): J. Neurosci., 7:88-100.
57. De Souza, E. B., and Battaglia, G.: In: Proc. NIH Conference on
    the Mechanisms of Physical and Emotional Stress, edited by P.
    W. Gold, and L. Loriaux, (in press).
58. Donald, R. A., Redekopp, C., Cameron, V., Nicholls, M. G.,
    Bolton, J., Livesey, J., Espiner, E. A., Rivier, J., and Vale,
    W. (1983): Endocrinology, 113:866-870.
59. Eaves, M., Thatcher-Britton, K., Rivier, J., Vale, W., and Koob,
    G. F. (1985): Peptides, 6:923-926.
60. Eberly, L. B., Dudley, C. A., and Moss, R. L. (1983): Peptides,
    4:837-841.

61. Ehlers, C. L., Henriksen, S. J., Wang, M., Rivier, J., Vale, W., and Bloom, F. E. (1983): Brain Res., 278:332-336.
62. Fehm, H. L., Voigt, K. H., Lang, R. E., and Pfeiffer, E. F. (1980): Exp. Brain Res., 39:229-234.
63. Feldman, S., Siegel, R. A., Weidenfeld, J., Conforti, N., and Melamed, E. (1983): Brain Res., 260:297-300.
64. Feldman, S., Melamed, E., Conforti, N., and Weidenfeld, J. (1984): Exp. Neurol., 85:661-666.
65. Feldman, S., Melamed, E., Conforti, N., and Weidenfeld, J. (1984): J. Neurosci. Res., 12:87-92.
66. Fellmann, D., Bugnon, C., and Gouger, A. (1982): Neurosci. Lett., 34:253-258.
67. Fink, G. (1981): Nature, 294:511-512.
68. Fischman, A. J., and Moldow, R. L. (1984): Life Sci., 35:1311-1319.
69. Fisher, L. A., and Brown, M. R. (1984): Brain Res., 296:41-47.
70. Furutani, Y., Morimoto, Y., Shibahara, S., Noda, M., Takahashi, H., Hirose, T., Asai, M., Inayama, S., Hayashida, H., Miyata, T., and Numa, S. (1983): Nature, 301:537-540.
71. Gagner, J.-P., and Drouin, J. (1985): Mol. Cell. Endocrinol., 40:25-32.
72. Gertz, B. J., Contreras, L. N., McComb, D. J., Kovacs, K., Tyrrell, J. B., and Dallman, M. F. (1987): Endocrinology, 120:381-388.
73. Gibbs, D. M., and Vale, W. (1982): Endocrinology, 111:1418-1420.
74. Gibbs, D. M., Stewart, R. D., Liu, J. H., Vale, W., Rivier, J., and Yen, S. S. C. (1982): J. Clin. Endocrinol. Metab., 55:1149-1152.
75. Gibbs, D. M., and Vale, W. (1983): Brain Res., 280:176-179.
76. Gibbs, D. M., Vale, W., Rivier, J., and Yen, S. S. C. (1984): Life Sci., 34:2245-2249.
77. Gibbs, D. M. (1985): Reg. Peptides, 12:273-277.
78. Gibson, A., Hart, S. L., and Patel, S. (1986): Neuropharmacology, 25:257-260.
79. Giguere, V., Labrie, F., Cote, J., Coy, D. H., Sueiras-Diaz, J., and Schally, A. V. (1982): Proc. Natl. Acad. Sci. USA, 79:3466-3469.
80. Giguere, V., and Labrie, F. (1982): Endocrinology, 111:1752-1754.
81. Giguere, V., Lefevre, G., and Labrie, F. (1982): Life Sci., 31:3057-3062.
82. Giguere, V., and Labrie, F. (1983): Biochem. Biophys. Res. Comm., 110:456-462.
83. Gold, P. W., Chrousos, G., Kellner, C., Post, R., Roy, A., Augerinos, P., Schulte, H., Oldfield, E., and Loriaux, D. L. (1984): Am. J. Psychiatry, 141:619-627.
84. Gold, P. W., and Chrousos, G. P. (1985): Psychoneuroendocrinology, 10:401-419.
85. Gosnell, B. A., Morley, J. E., and Levine, A. S. (1983): Pharmacol. Biochem. Behav., 19:771-775.
86. Graf, M. V., Kastin, A. J., and Fischman, A. J. (1985): Proc. Soc. Exp. Biol. Med., 179:303-308.
87. Guillemin, R., and Rosenberg, B. (1955): Endocrinology, 57:599-607.

88. Guillemin, R., Schally, A. V., Lipscomb, H. S., Andersen, R. N., and Long, J. M. (1962): Endocrinology, 70:471-477.
89. Guillemin, R., Cohn, M., and Melneckuk, T. (1983): Neural Modulation of Immunity. Raven Press, New York.
90. Hargrave, B. Y., and Rose, J. C. (1986): Am. Physiol. Soc., 422-427.
91. Hashimoto, K., Ohno, N., Murakami, K., Kageyama, J., Aoki, Y., and Takahara, J. (1982): Endocrinol. Japan, 29:383-388.
92. Hashimoto, K., Ono, N., Hattori, T., Suemaru, S., Inoue, H., Kawada, Y., Kageyama, J., and Ota, Z. (1986): Endocrinol. Japan, 33:95-103.
93. Hauger, R. L. (1986): Abst. Endocrine Soc., 640.
94. Hayes, A. G., and Stewart, B. R. (1985): Eur. J. Pharmacol., 116:75-79.
95. Hedge, G. A., and Smelik, P. G. (1968): Science, 159:891-892.
96. Heisler, S., Hook, V. Y. H., and Axelrod, J. (1983): Biochem. Pharmacol., 32:1295-1299.
97. Herkenham, M. and McLean, S. (1986): Quantitative Receptor Autoradiography. Alan R. Liss, Inc.
98. Hermus, A., Raemaekers, J. M. M., Pieters, G. F. F. M., Bartelink, A. K. M., Smals, A. G. H., and Kloppenborg, P. W. C. (1983): Lancet, (April 2) 776.
99. Hermus, A., Raemaekers, J. M. M., Pieters, G. F. F. M., Bartelink, A. K. M., Smals, A. G. H., and Kloppenborg, P. W. C. (1983): Lancet (July 9) 112.
100. Hermus, A. R. M. M., Pieters, G. F. F. M., Pesman, G. J., Buys, W. C. A. M., Smals, A. G. H., Benraad, T. J., and Kloppenborg, P. W. C. (1984): Clin. Endocrinol., 21:589-595.
101. Hillhouse, E. W., Burden, J., and Jones, M. T. (1975): Neuroendocrinology, 17:1-11.
102. Hoffman, A. R., Ceda, G., and Reisine, T. D. (1985): J. Neurosci., 5:234-242.
103. Hokfelt, T., Fahrenkrug, J., Tatemoto, K., Mutt, V., Werner, S., Hulting, A.-L., Terenius, L., and Chang, K. J. (1983): Proc. Natl. Acad. Sci. USA, 80:895-898.
104. Holmes, M. C., Di Renzo, G., Beckford, U., Gillham, B., and Jones, M. T. (1982): J. Endocrinol., 93:151-160.
105. Holmes, M. C., Antoni, F. A., and Szentendrei, T. (1984): Neuroendocrinology, 39:162-169.
106. Holmes, M. C., Antoni, F. A., Catt, K. J., and Aguilera, G. (1986): Neuroendocrinology, 43:245-251.
107. Holsboer, F., Bardeleben, U. V., Gerken, A., Stalla, G. K., and Muller, O. A. (1984): New Eng. J. Med., 311:1127.
108. Holsboer, F., Muller, O. A., Doerr, H. G., Sippell, W. G., Stalla, G. K., Gerken, A., Steiger, A., Boll, E., and Benkert, O. (1984): Psychoneuroendocrinology, 9:147-160.
109. Hook, V. Y. H., Heisler, S., Sabol, S. L., and Axelrod, J. (1982): Biochem. Biophys. Res. Comm., 106:1364-1371.
110. Hook, V. Y. H., Heisler, S., and Axelrod, J. (1982): Proc. Natl. Acad. Sci. USA, 79:6220-6224.
111. Hotta, M., Shibasaki, T., Masuda, A., Imaki, T., Demura, H., Ling, N., and Shizume, K. (1986): J. Clin. Endocrinol. Metab., 62:319-324.
112. Insel, T. R., Aloi, J. A., Goldstein, D., Wood, J. H., and Jimerson, D. C. (1984): Life Sci., 34:1873-1878.

113. Iyengar, S., Kim, H. S., and Wood, P. L. (1986): J. Pharmacol. Exp. Ther., 238:429-436.
114. Jones, M. T., and Hillhouse, E. W. (1976): J. Steroid Biochem., 7:1189-1202.
115. Jones, M. T., Hillhouse, E. W., and Burden, J. (1976): J. Endocrinol., 69:1-10.
116. Jones, M. T., Birmingham, N., Gillham, B., Holmes, M., and Smith, T. (1979): Clin. Endocrinol., 10:203-205.
117. Kalin, N. H., Gonder, J. C., and Shelton, S. E. (1983): Peptides, 4:221-223.
118. Kalin, N. H., Shelton, S. E., Kraemer, G. W., and McKinney, W. T. (1983): Peptides, 4:217-220.
119. Kalivas, P. W., Duffy, P., and Latimer, L. G. J. Pharmacol. Exp. Ther., (in press).
120. Katakami, H., Arimura, A., and Frohman, L. A. (1985): Neuroendocrinology, 41:390-393.
121. Kile, J. P., and Turner, B. B. (1985): Experientia 41:1123-1127.
122. Kilts, C. D., Bissette, G., Krishnan, K. R. R., Smith, M.A., Chappel, P., and Nemeroff, C. B. (1986): In: Hormones and Depression, edited by U. Halbreich and R. M. Rose. Raven Press, New York.
123. Knepel, W., Homolka, L., Vlaskovska, M., and Nutto, D. (1984): Neuroendocrinology, 38:344-350.
124. Koob, G. F., Swerdlow, N., Seeligson, M., Eaves, M., Sutton, R., Rivier, J., and Vale, W. (1984): Neuroendocrinology, 39:459-464.
125. Koob, G. F. (1984): In: Perspectives on Behavioral Medicine: Neuroendocrine Control and Behavior, edited by R. M. Williams. Academic Press, New York.
126. Koob, G. F., and Thatcher-Britton, K. (1984): In: Proc. First Int. Symposium on Endocoids. A.R. Liss.
127. Koob, G. F., and Bloom, F. E. (1985): Fed. Proc. 44:220-222.
128. Kraicer, J., Gajewski, T. C., and Moore, B. C. (1985): Neuroendocrinology, 41:363-373.
129. Krieger, D. T., and Liotta, A. S. (1979): Science, 205:366-372.
130. Lau, S. H., Rivier, J., Vale, W., Kaiser, E. T., and Kezdy, F. J. (1983): Proc. Natl. Acad. Sci. USA, 80:7070-7074.
131. Levine, A. S., Rogers, B., Kneip, J., Grace, M., and Morley, J. E. (1983): Life Sci., 22:337-339.
132. Linton, E. A., Tilders, F. J. H., Hodgkinson, S., Berkenbosch, F., Vermes, I., and Lowry, P. J. (1985): Endocrinology, 116:966-970.
133. Liposits, Z., Lengvari, I., Vigh, S., Schally, A. V., and Flerko, B. (1983): Peptides, 4:941-953.
134. Liposits, Z., Sherman, D., Phelix, C., and Paull, W. K. (1986): Histochemistry, 84:95-106.
135. Liposits, Z., Phelix, C., and Paull, W. K. (1986): Histochemistry, 85:201-205.
136. Litvin, Y., PasMantier, R., Fleischer, N., and Erlichman, J. (1984): J. Biol. Chem., 259:10296-10302.
137. Litvin, Y., Leiser, M., Fleischer, N., and Erlichman, J. (1986): Endocrinology, 119:737-745.
138. Liu, J. H., Muse, K., Contreras, P., Gibbs, D., Vale, W., Rivier, J., and Yen, S. S. C. (1983): J. Clin. Endocrinol. Metab., 57:1087-1089.

139. Loeffler, J. Ph., Kley, N., Pittius, C. W., and Hollt, V.
     (1985): Neurosci. Lett., 62:383-387.
140. MacIsaac, R. J., Bell, R. J., McDougall, J. G., Tregear, G. W.,
     Wang, X., and Wintour, E. M. (1985): J. Dev. Physiol.,
     7:329-338.
141. Maiewski, S. F., Larscheid, P., Cook, J. M., and Mueller, G. P.
     (1985): Endocrinology, 117:474-480.
142. Maser-Gluth, C., Toygar, A., and Vecsei, P. (1984): Life Sci.,
     35:879-884.
143. Merchenthaler, I., Vigh, S., Petrusz, P., and Schally, A. V.
     (1983): Peptides, 5:295-305.
144. Merchenthaler, I., Hynes, M. A., Vigh, S., Schally, A. V., and
     Petrusz, P. (1984): Neuroendocrinology, 39:296-306.
145. Mezey, E., Kiss, J. Z., Skirboll, L. R., Goldstein, M., and
     Axelrod, J. (1984): Nature, 310:140-141.
146. Millan, M. A., Jacobowitz, D. M., Hauger, R. L., Catt, K. J., and
     Aguilera, G. (1986): Proc. Natl. Acad. Sci. USA,
     83:1921-1925.
147. Moga, M. M., and Gray, T. S. (1985): J. Comp. Neurol.,
     241:275-284.
148. Morley, J. E., and Levine, A. S. (1982): Life Sci.,
     31:1459-1464.
149. Morley, J. E., Levine, A. S., Gosnell, B. A., and Krahn, D. D.
     (1985): Brain Res. Bull., 14:511-519.
150. Mueller, E. A., Murphy, D. L., and Sunderland, T. (1985): J.
     Clin. Endocrinol. Metab., 61:1179-1184.
151. Muller, O. A., Hartwimmer, J., Hauer, A., Kaliebe, T., Schopohl,
     J., Stalla, G. K., and von Werder, K. (1986): Psychoneuroendo-
     crinology, 11:49-60.
152. Murakami, K., Hashimoto, K., and Ota, Z. (1984): Neuroendocri-
     nology, 39:49-53.
153. Murakami, K., Hashimoto, K., and Ota, Z. (1985): Neuroendocri-
     nology, 41:7-12.
154. Murakami, K., Hashimoto, K., and Ota, Z. (1985): Acta
     Endocrinologica, 109:32-36.
155. Murburg, M. M., Paly, D., Wilkinson, C. W., Veith, R. C., Malas,
     K. L., and Dorsa, D. M. (1986): Life Sci., 39:373-381.
156. Nakagami, Y., Suda, T., Yajima, F., Ushiyama, T., Tomori, N.,
     Sumitomo, T., Demura, H., and Shizume, K. (1986): Brain Res.,
     386:232-236.
157. Nakane, T., Audhya, T., Kanie, N., and Hollander, C. S. (1985):
     Proc. Natl. Acad. Sci. USA, 82:1247-1251.
158. Nemeroff, C. B., Widerlov, E., Bissette, G., Walleus, H.,
     Karlsson, I, Eklund, K., Kilts, C. D., Loosen, P. T., and
     Vale, W. (1984): Science, 226:1342-1344.
159. Nicholson, S., Lin, J.-H., Mahmoud, S., Campbell, E., Gillham,
     B., and Jones, M. (1985): Neuroendocrinology, 40:217-224.
160. Nikolarakis, K. E., Almeida, O. F. X., and Herz, A. (1986):
     Brain Res., 377:388-390.
161. Nikolarakis, K. E., Almeida, O. F. X., and Herz, A. (1986):
     Brain Res., 399:152-155.
162. Ono, N., Lumpkin, M. D., Samson, W. K., McDonald, J. K., and
     McCann, S. M. (1984): Life Sci., 35:1117-1123.
163. Ono, N., Bedran de Castro, J. C., and McCann, S. M. (1985):
     Proc. Natl. Acad. Sci. USA, 82:3528-3531.

164. Ono, N., Samson, W. K., McDonald, J. K., Lumpkin, M.D., Bedran de Castro, J. C., and McCann, S. M. (1985): Proc. Natl. Acad. Sci. USA, 82:7787-7790.
165. Palkovits, M., and Brownstein, M. J. (1983): In: Brain Microdissection Techniques, edited by A. C. Cuello (IBRO Handbook Series: Methods in the Neurosciences, Volume 2), pp. 1-36. John Wiley & Sons.
166. Patthy, M., Schlesinger, D. H., Horvath, J., Mason-Garcia, M., Szoke, B., and Schally, A. V. (1986): Proc. Natl. Acad. Sci. USA, 83:2969-2973.
167. Pechnick, R. N., George, R., Lee, R. J., and Poland, R. E. (1986): Life Sci., 38:291-296.
168. Perrin, M. H., Haas, Y., Rivier, J. E., and Vale, W. W. (1986): Endocrinology, 118:1171-1179.
169. Peterfreund, R. A., and Vale, W. W. (1983): Endocrinology, 112:1275-1278.
170. Petrusz, P., Merchenthaler, I., Maderdrut, J. L., Vigh, S., and Schally, A. V. (1983): Proc. Natl. Acad. Sci. USA, 80:1721-1725.
171. Petrusz, P., Merchenthaler, I., Ordronneau, P., Maderdrut, J. L., Vigh, S., and Schally, A. V. (1984): Peptides, 5(Suppl. 1):71-78.
172. Petrusz, P., Merchenthaler, I., Maderdrut, J. L., and Heita, P. V. (1985): Fed. Proc., 44:229-235.
173. Pfeiffer, A., Herz, A., Loriaux, D. L., and Pfeiffer, D. G. (1985): Endocrinology, 116:2688-2690.
174. Piekut, D. T., and Joseph, S. A. (1985): Peptides, 6:873-882.
175. Piekut, D. T., and Joseph, S. A. (1986): Peptides, 7:891-898.
176. Pieters, G. F. F. M., Hermus, A. R. M. M., Smals, A. G. H., Bartelink, A. K. M., Benraad, Th. J., and Kloppenborg, P. W. C. (1983): J. Clin. Endocrinol. Metab., 57:513-516.
177. Plotsky, P. M., and Vale, W. (1984): Endocrinology, 114:164-1169.
178. Plotsky, P. M., Bruhn, T. O., and Vale, W. (1984): Endocrinology, 115:1639-1641.
179. Plotsky, P. M., Bruhn, T. O., and Otto, S. (1984): Endocrinology, 116:1669-1671.
180. Plotsky, P. M. (1985): Fed. Proc., 44:207-213.
181. Plotsky, P. M., Bruhn, T. O., and Vale, W. (1985): Endocrinology, 117:323-329.
182. Plotsky, P. M., Otto, S., and Sapolsky, R. M. (1986): Endocrinology, 119:1126-1130.
183. Plotsky, P. M. (1986): Reg. Peptides, 16:235-242.
184. Powers, R. E., De Souza, E. B., Walker, L. C., Vale, W. W., Price, D. L., and Young, W. S. (1986): Soc. Neurosci. Abstr. 12:157.5.
185. Pradier, P., Davicco, M. J., Safwate, A., Tournaire, C., Dalle, M., Barlet, J. P., and Delost, P. (1986): Acta Endocrinologica, 111:93-100.
186. Proulx-Ferland, L., Labrie, F., Dumont, D., and Cote, J. (1982): Science, 217:62-63.
187. Radnai, Z., and Endroczi, E. (1979): Acta Physiol. Acad. Sci. Hung., 54:129-139.
188. Redekopp, C. A., Livesey, J. H., and Donald, R. A. (1985): Horm. Metabol. Res., 17:646-649.

189. Redekopp, C., Livesey, J. H., Sadler, W., and Donald, R. A.
     (1986): J. Endocrinol., 108:309-312.
190. Reisine, T., and Hoffman, A. (1983): Biochem. Biophys. Res.
     Comm., 111:919-925.
191. Reisine, T., Rougon, G., Barbet, J., and Affolter, H.-U. (1985):
     Proc. Natl. Acad. Sci. USA, 82:8261-8265.
192. Ritchie, J. C., Owens, M. J., O'Connor, L., Kegelmeyer, A. E.,
     Walker, J. T., Stanley, M., Bissette, G., and Nemeroff, C. B.
     (1986): Soc. Neuroscience Abstr., 12:286.5.
193. Rivier, C., Rivier, J., and Vale, W. (1982): Science,
     218:377-378.
194. Rivier, C., Brownstein, M., Spiess, J., Rivier, J., and Vale, W.
     (1982): Endocrinology, 110:272-278.
195. Rivier, C., and Vale, W. (1983): Nature, 305:325-327.
196. Rivier, C., and Vale, W. (1983): Endocrinology, 113:939-942.
197. Rivier, J., Rivier, C., and Vale, W. (1984): Science,
     224:889-891.
198. Rivier, C., and Vale, W. (1984): Endocrinology, 114:914-921.
199. Rivier, C., and Vale, W. (1984): Endocrinology, 114:2409-2411.
200. Rivier, C., Rivier, J., Mormede, P., and Vale, W. (1984):
     Endocrinology, 115:882-886.
201. Rivier, C., Bruhn, T., and Vale, W. (1984): J. Pharmacol. Exp.
     Ther., 229:127-131.
202. Rivier, C., and Vale, W. (1985): Fed. Proc., 44:189-195.
203. Rivier, C., and Vale, W. (1985): Endocrinology, 117:2478-2482.
204. Rivier, C., and Vale, W. (1985): In: Vasopressin, edited by
     Schrier, R. W., pp. 181-188. Raven Press, New York.
205. Rivier, C., and Vale, W. (1985): J. Clin. Invest., 75:689-694.
206. Rivier, C., and Rivier, J., and Vale, W. (1986): Science,
     231:607-609.
207. Rock, J. P., Oldfield, E. H., Schulte, H. M., Gold, P. W.,
     Kornblith, P. L., Loriaux, L., and Chrousos, G. P. (1984):
     Brain Res., 323:365-368.
208. Roth, K. A., Katz, R. J., Sibel, M., Mefford, I. N., Barchas, J.
     D., and Carroll, B. J. (1981): Life Sci., 28:2389-2394.
209. Roth, K. A., Weber, E., Barchas, J. D., Chang, D., and Change,
     J.-K. (1983): Science, 219:189-191.
210. Ruckebusch, Y., and Malbert, C. H. (1986): Life Sci.,
     38:929-934.
211. Saffran, M., and Schally, A. V. (1955): Can. J. Biochem.
     Physiol., 33:408-415.
212. Sakakura, M., Yoshioka, M., Kobayashi, M., and Takebe, K.
     (1981): Neuroendocrinology, 32:38-41.
213. Sapolsky, R. M., and Meaney, M. J. (1986): Brain Res. Rev.,
     11:65-76.
214. Sasaki, A., Liotta, A. S., Luckey, M. M., Margioris, A. N., Suda,
     T., and Krieger, D. T. (1984): J. Clin. Endocrinol. Metab.,
     59:812-814.
215. Saunders, W. S., and Thornhill, J. A. (1986): Peptides,
     7:597-601.
216. Sawchenko, P. E., Swanson, L. W., and Vale, W. W. (1984): J.
     Neuroscience, 4:1118-1129.
217. Sawchenko, P. E., Swanson, L. W., and Vale, W. W. (1984): Proc.
     Natl. Acad. Sci. USA, 81:1883-1887.

218. Sawchenko, P. E., and Swanson, L. W. (1985): Fed. Proc., 44:221-227.
219. Schally, A. V., Anderson, R. N., Lipscomb, H. S., Long, J. M., and Guillemin, R. (1960): Nature, 188:1192-1193.
220. Schally, A. V., Lipscomp, H. S., and Guillemin, R. (1962): Endocrinology, 71:161-173.
221. Schteingart, D. E., Lloyd, R. V., Akil, H., Chandler, W. F., Ibarra-Perez, G., Rosen, S. G., and Ogletree, R. (1986): J. Clin. Endocrinol. Metab., 63:770-775.
222. Schulte, H. M., Chrousos, G. P., Oldfield, E. H., Gold, P. W., Cutler, G. B., Jr., and Loriaux, D. L. (1982): J. Clin. Endocrinol. Metab., 55:810-812.
223. Schulte, H. M., Chrousos, G. P., Gold, P. W., Booth, J. D., Oldfield, E. H., Cutler, G. B., Jr., and Loriaux, D. L. (1985): J. Clin. Invest., 75:1781-1785.
224. Schwartz, J., Billestrup, N., Perrin, M., Rivier, J., and Vale, W. (1986): Endocrinology, 119:2376-2382.
225. Seltzer, A. M., Donoso, A. O., and Podesta, E. (1986): Physiol. Behav., 36:251-255.
226. Sherman, J. E., and Kalin, N. H. (1986): Life Sci., 39:433-441.
227. Shibahara, T., Morimoto, Y., Furutani, Y., Notake, M., Takahashi, H., Shimizu, S., Horikawa, N., and Numa, S. (1983): EMBO J., 2:775-779.
228. Siggins, G. R., Gruol, D., Aldenhoff, J., and Pittman, Q. (1985): Fed. Proc., 44:237-242.
229. Sirinathsinghji, D. J. S., Rees, L. H., Rivier, J., and Vale, W. (1983): Nature, 305:232-235.
230. Sirinathsinghji, D. J. S. (1986): Brain Res., 375:49-56.
231. Skofitsch, G., Zamir, N., Helke, C. J., Savitt, J. M., and Jacobowitz, D. M. (1985): Peptides, 6:307-318.
232. Smith, E. M., Morrill, A. C., Meyer, W. J., III, and Blalock, J. E. (1986): Nature, 322:881-882.
233. Smith, M. A., Bissette, G., Slotkin, T. A., Knight, D. L., and Nemeroff, C. B. (1986): Endocrinology, 118:1997-2001.
234. Smythe, G. A., Bradshaw, J. E., and Vining, R. F. (1983): Endocrinology, 113:1062-1070.
235. Spiess, J., Rivier, J., Rivier, C., and Vale, W. (1981): Proc. Natl. Acad. Sci. USA, 78:6517-6521.
236. Spinedi, E., and Rodriguez, G. (1986): Endocrinology, 119:1397-1402.
237. Suda, T., Tomori, N., Tozawa, F., Demura, H., Shizume, K., Mouri, T., Miura, Y., and Sasano, N. (1984): J. Clin. Endocrinol. Metab., 58:919-924.
238. Suda, T., Yajima, F., Tomori, N., Demura, H., and Shizume, K. (1985): Life Sci., 37:1499-1505.
239. Suda, T., Tomori, N., Yajima, F., Sumitomo, T., Nakagami, Y., Ushiyama, T., Demura, H., and Shizume, K. (1985): J. Clin. Invest., 76:2026-2029.
240. Suda, T., Yajima, F., Tomori, N., Sumitomo, T., Nakagami, Y., Ushiyama, T., Demura, H., and Shizume, K. (1986): Endocrinology, 118:459-461.
241. Suda, T., Yajima, F., Tomori, N., Sumitomo, T., Nakagami, Y., Ushiyama, T., Demura, H., and Shizume, K. (1987): Life Sci., 40:673-677.

242. Suemaru, S., Hashimoto, K., and Ota, Z. (1985): Acta Med.
      Okayama, 39:463-470.
243. Sutton, R. E., Koob, G. F., Le Moal, M., Rivier, J., and Vale, W.
      (1982): Nature, 297:331-333.
244. Swanson, L. W., Sawchenko, P. E., Rivier, J., and Vale, W. W.
      (1983): Neuroendocrinology, 36:165-186.
245. Swerdlow, N. R., and Koob, G. F. (1985): Pharmacol. Biochem.
      Behav., 23:303-307.
246. Swerdlow, N. R., Geyer, M. A., Vale, W. W., and Koob, G. F.
      (1986): Psychopharmacology, 88:147-152.
247. Tache, Y., Goto, Y., Gunion, M. W., Vale, W., Rivier, J., and
      Brown, M. (1983): Science, 222:935-937.
248. Tate, P. W., Newell, D. C., Cook, E. E., Martinson, D. R., and
      Hagen, T. C. (1983): Horm. Metabol. Res., 15:342-346.
249. Tilders, F. J. H., Berkenbosch, F., Vermes, I., Linton, E. A.,
      and Smelik, P. G. (1985): Fed. Proc., 44:155-160.
250. Tonon, M. C., Cuet, P., Lamacz, M., Jegou, S., Cote, J., Gouteux,
      L., Ling, N., Pelletier, G., and Vaudry, H. (1985): Gen.
      Comp. Endocrinol., 61:438-445.
251. Udelsman, R., Harwood, J. P., Millan, M. A., Chrousos, G. P.,
      Goldstein, D. S., Zimlichman, R., Catt, K. J., and Aguilera,
      G. (1986): Nature, 319:147-150.
252. Udelsam, R., Gallucci, W. T., Bacher, J., Loriaux, D. L.,
      Chrousos, G. P. (1986): Peptides, 7:465-471.
253. Upton, G. V., and Corbin, A. (1975): Experientia, 31:249-250.
254. Vacca, M., Cerrito, F., and Preziosi, P. (1983): Arch. Int.
      Pharmacodyn., 263:328-330.
255. Vale, W., Spiess, J., Rivier, C., and Rivier, J. (1981):
      Science, 213:1394-1397.
256. Vale, W., Rivier, C., Brown, M., Spiess, J., Koob, G., Swanson,
      L., Bilezikjian, L., Bloom, F., and Rivier, J. (1983): In:
      Recent Progress in Hormone Research, vol. 39, pp. 245-270.
      Academic Press, Inc.
257. Vale, W. Vaughan, J., Smith, M., Yamamoto, G., Rivier, J., and
      Rivier, C. (1983): Endocrinology, 113:1121-1131.
258. Valentino, R. J., Foote, S. L., and Aston-Jones, G. (1983):
      Brain Res., 270:363-367.
259. Valentino, R. J., Martin, D. L., and Suzuki, M. (1986):
      Neuropharmacology, 25:603-610.
260. Valentino, R. J., and Foote, S. L. In: Neural and Endocrine
      Peptides and Receptors, edited by Moody, M., pp. 101-119.
      Plenum (in press).
261. Van Loon, G. R., Scapagnini, U., Moberg, G. P., and Ganong, W. F.
      (1971): Endocrinology, 89:1464-1469.
262. Veldhuis, H. D., and De Wied, D. (1984): Pharmacol. Biochem.
      Behav., 21:707-713.
263. Weiss, S. R. B., Post, R. M., Gold, P. W., Chrousos, G.,
      Sullivan, T. L., Walker, D., and Pert, A. (1986): Brain Res.,
      372:345-351.
264. Whitnall, M. H., Mezey, E., and Gainer, H. (1985): Nature,
      317:248-250.
265. Widerlov, E., Ekman, R., and Wahlestedt, C. (1986): Abstr. 15th
      Coll. Int. Neuro-Psychopharmacol., 207.
266. Widmaier, E. P., and Dallman, M. F. (1984): Endocrinology,
      115:2368-2374.

267. Woloski, B. M. R. N. J., Smith, E. M., Meyer, W. J., III, and Fuller, G. M., and Blalock, J. E. (1985): Science, 230:1035-1037.
268. Wynn, P. C., Aguilera, G., Morell, J., and Catt, K. J. (1983): Biochem. Biophys. Res. Comm., 110:602-608.
269. Wynn, P. C., Hauger, R. L., Holmes, M. C., Millan, M. A., Catt, K. J., and Aguilera, G. (1984): Peptides, 5:1077-1084.
270. Yajima, F., Suda, T., Tomori, N., Sumitomo, T., Nakagami, Y., Ushiyama, T., Demura, H., and Shizume, K. (1986): Life Sci., 39:181-186.
271. Yasuda, N., Yasuda, Y., Aizawa, T., Maruta, S., and Greer, M. A. (1984): Acta Endocrinologica, 106:158-167.
272. Young, E. A., and Akil, H. (1985): Endocrinology, 117:23-30.

The Hypothalamic-Pituitary-Adrenal Axis:
Physiology, Pathophysiology, and Psychiatric
Implications, edited by A.F. Schatzberg and
C.B. Nemeroff. Raven Press, Ltd., New York
© 1988.

ANALYTICAL AND METHODOLOGICAL CONSIDERATIONS

IN THE STUDY OF THE HPA AXIS

Clinton D. Kilts, Karen L. Johnson and James C. Ritchie

Departments of Psychiatry and Pharmacology
Duke University Medical Center
Durham, North Carolina 27710

The physiology and pathophysiology of the hypothalamic–pituitary–adrenal (HPA) axis has become an increasing focus of both preclinical and clinical research. Studies of the mechanisms of regulation of the output of each component of this axis has been greatly aided by the recent use of molecular probes and model cell systems (25,6). It has become increasingly clear that the output of each component of the axis reflects the integrated, net actions of a multitude of complementary regulators including classical neurotransmitters, neuropeptides and the immune system (44) and that the activity in the HP axis is also tightly regulated by feedback mechanisms ranging from long–loop to ultra–short mechanisms (33). This discussion will concern the application of various analytical techniques and methods to the study of each of these components; the neurochemical anatomy of the hypothalamus, the radioimmunoassay (RIA) of plasma adrenocorticotropin hormone (ACTH) and the quantification of plasma dexamethasone by mass fragmentography. Emphasis will be on specific aspects of the analytical or methodological challenge posed by each problem as they relate to the design of the technique applied.

NEUROCHEMICAL ANATOMY OF THE HYPOTHALAMUS

Although extrahypothalamic brain structures, particularly limbic, are thought to modulate the activity of the HPA axis (18) the hypothalamus is generally regarded to be the peak of this functional cascade. As is typical of the organization of limbic brain structures, the hypothalamus is actually an assembly of biochemically, anatomically and functionally heterogeneous nuclear groups (27,41). The neurochemical anatomy of the hypothalamus, as defined by micromapping the distribution of norepinephrine, epinephrine, dopamine and CRF in discrete component nuclei is illustrated in Table 1. The hypothalamic nuclei of interest were micropunch dissected from coronal slices of the rat brain (41,43) and catecholamines and CRF were quantitated by on-line trace enrichment HPLC with electrochemical detection (30) and radioimmunoassay (14), respectively. The heterogeneous distribution of norepinephrine, epinephrine, dopamine and CRF supports a differential

role of these neuroregulators in modulating or mediating the output of
discrete hypothalamic nuclei. The CRF-containing neurons projecting
from the parvocellular subdivision of the PVN to the external zone of
the median eminence constitutes the major mechanism of central
regulation of the pituitary-adrenal axis (35,11). The topographic
distribution of CRF in the PVN and median eminence (Table 1) is
consistent with this functional organization, though the appreciable
amount of CRF in other hypothalamic nuclei is consistent with the
widespread role of this system in regulating diverse neuroendocrine,
central autonomic and behavioral processes (47).

Table 1

NEUROCHEMICAL ANATOMY OF THE RAT HYPOTHALAMUS

Nuclei	Catecholamines[a]			CRF-like[b] immunoreactivity
	Norepinephrine	Epinephrine	Dopamine	
Paraventricular	73.7 ± 5.5	3.6 ± 0.36	7.4 ± 0.23	498 ± 44
Periventricular (tuberal)	26.3 ± 2.5	0.78 ± 0.06	3.4 ± 0.51	316 ± 15
Dorsomedial	26.1 ± 2.0	0.98 ± 0.25	2.7 ± 0.19	114 ± 7
Ventromedial	12.9 ± 0.90	0.27 ± 0.02	1.7 ± 0.10	97 ± 15
Arcuate	21.5 ± 0.80	0.73 ± 0.06	11.4 ± 1.9	285 ± 46
Median eminence	-	-	-	5054 ± 674
Anterior	10.0 ± 0.79	n.d.[c]	1.6 ± 0.07	93 ± 7
Lateral	11.6 ± 0.88	0.37 ± 0.04	1.1 ± 0.17	121 ± 14
Supraoptic	-	-	-	133 ± 23
Suprachiasmatic	-	-	-	162 ± 36
Medial preoptic	23.8 ± 2.2	0.98 ± 0.18	3.4 ± 0.68	143 ± 11
Lateral preoptic	16.3 ± 2.1	n.d.	1.7 ± 0.18	86 ± 6

[a]Values represent the mean ± SEM of 5 or 6 determinations expressed as catecholamine/mg
protein

[b]Values represent the mean ± SEM of 5-10 determinations expressed as pg CRF-LI/mg protein

[c]n.d. = not detectable (< 10 pg/sample)

　　　If anatomical distribution reflects the functional organization of
neurotransmitter systems then a comparison of the topographic
distribution of catecholamines in the hypothalamus may indicate their
relative role in modulating the activity of CRF-containing neurons in
the PVN. The striking concentration of norepinephrine and epinephrine
in the PVN, relative to other hypothalamic nuclei, (Table 1), suggests a
critical role in regulating the HPA axis. Considerable functional
evidence supports the role of noradrenergic neurons in regulating the
functional output of CRF-containing cells (20,47) though it is unclear
as to whether the influence of norepinephrine is exerted at somato-
dendritic or nerve terminal sites of action, or both.

ROLE OF EPINEPHRINE-CONTAINING NEURONS IN THE CENTRAL REGULATION
OF THE HPA AXIS

Of the neuronal systems in the CNS utilizing catecholamines for synaptic transmission, those containing epinephrine represent by far the minority. However, epinephrine (EPI) neurons appear to be organized into discrete populations focally innervating circumscribed projection fields from medullary localized cell bodies (24). In addition to the dense localization of EPI in the PVN (Table 1), both functional and anatomical evidence supports a key role for EPI neurons in regulating the activity of CRF neurons emanating from the PVN. The pharmacological inhibition of phenylethanolamine-N-methyltransferase (PNMT), the terminal enzyme catalyzing the biosynthesis of EPI (5), produces a significant increase in the number of CRF-immunopositive cells in the PVN (37), suggesting a tonic inhibitory influence of EPI on CRF synthesis. Immunocytochemical studies indicate that PNMT-immunopositive axon terminals establish direct synaptic connections with somata, dendrites and spinous structures of CRF-immunoreactive neurons in the PVN (1,34). In a more thorough examination of the functional significance of EPI neurons in the CNS and their association with CRF neurons, we attempted to estimate, by biochemical turnover techniques, the activity of EPI neurons innervating the PVN and other hypothalamic as well as telencephalic or medullary nuclei. The rate of turnover or utilization of EPI in neuronal populations innervating discrete brain nuclei was determined from the rate of decline of EPI concentration with time following the administration of the PNMT inhibitor LY134046 (19). The rate of depletion of EPI in the hypothalamic nuclei examined following the administration of LY134046 followed first order kinetics (Fig. 1). The rate constants calculated from the slopes of the LY134046-induced depletion of EPI, the time required for a 50% depletion of EPI ($t_{1/2}$) and the estimated rate of EPI synthesis in the hypothalamic nuclei examined are summarized in Table 2. A comparison of the rate constants for the decline of EPI indicated a dissimilar estimated activity of EPI neuronal populations innervating discrete hypothalamic nuclei with the fastest and slowest rates observed in the arcuate nucleus and pretuberal periventricular nucleus, respectively. In general, the estimated rate of impulse activity of hypothalamic EPI neurons exceeded that of brain norepinephrine neurons and, with the exception of mesocortical and some populations of mesolimbic neurons, that of dopamine neurons (31). These results have important implications for the physiology of EPI neurotransmission in the hypothalamus. First, the influence of EPI as a neurotransmitter in the hypothalamus apparently varies between the component nuclear groups. Secondly, examination of the dynamics of hypothalamic EPI neurons elevates their relative functional role as neurotransmitters beyond that predicted from content alone. The next phase of these experiments involves the determination of the influence of manipulating the functional activity of the hypothalamic-pituitary system (e.g. adrenalectomy, steroid supplementation) on the estimated activity of EPI neurons innervating the PVN relative to other EPI neuronal populations.

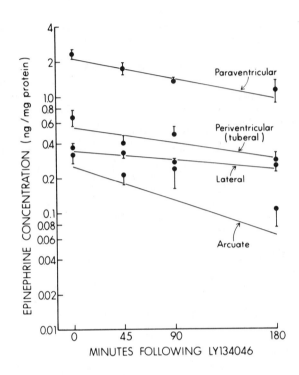

FIG 1. Semilogarithmic plot of the
concentration of epinephrine in
discrete hypothalamic nuclei vs.
time following the administration of
LY134046.

CRF AUTORECEPTORS IN THE PVN: COUPLING TO THE ADENYLATE CYCLASE SECOND MESSENGER SYSTEM

The receptor-mediated actions of CRF on ACTH release from
corticotrophs in the anterior pituitary is mediated by an activation of
adenylate cyclase and resulting increases in cAMP formation (21,2). The
coupling of CRF receptors to this second messenger system has also been
demonstrated in the CNS. CRF has been shown to produce a concentration-
and guanyl nucleotide-dependent increase in adenylate cyclase activity
in homogenates of the frontoparietal cortex, olfactory bulb, cerebellum,
midbrain, hippocampus and amygdala but not pons or spinal cord (49,3,7).
Biochemical and anatomical evidence indicates that CRF-synthesizing
neurons in the PVN may autoregulate their functional activity via an
ultrashort feedback mechanism. An appreciable density of CRF receptors
in the PVN has been demonstrated by in vitro quantitative
autoradiography (15) and electron microscope immunohistochemical
analyses indicate that CRF-containing axons emanating from the PVN

Table 2

KINETIC PARAMETERS DESCRIBING THE DYNAMICS OF EPINEPHRINE-CONTAINING NEURONAL POPULATIONS

INNERVATING DISCRETE HYPOTHALAMIC NUCLEI

Nuclei	Epinephrine Concentration ng/mg protein	Rate constant (k)[a] $(1/h)$	$t_{1/2}$[b]	Synthesis Rate (ng EPI/mg protein/h)
Paraventricular	2.4 ± 0.22	-0.278 ± 0.06	2.50	0.653
Periventricular				
Tuberal	0.67 ± 0.10	-0.208 ± 0.09	3.33	0.140
Pretuberal	0.60 ± 0.05	-0.099 ± 0.08	6.99	0.061
Lateral	0.37 ± 0.04	-0.130 ± 0.05	5.35	0.048
Dorsomedial	0.90 ± 0.06	-0.108 ± 0.08	6.41	0.097
Arcuate	0.32 ± 0.05	-0.449 ± 0.17	1.54	0.144

[a] k ($\pm$ S.E.E.) was calculated from the slope obtained by computing a least squares regression analysis of the common logarithm of the epinephrine concentration found 0, 0.75, 1.5 and 3 hr after LY 134046 (40 mg/kg, i.p.).

[b] time required for a 50% depletion of epinephrine

branch into axon collaterals which establish axo-somatic synapses on CRF-immunopositive neurons in the PVN (33). In a further application of micropunch dissection techniques to the study of the regulation of the HPA axis we sought to determine if CRF "autoreceptors" in the PVN were similarly coupled to the adenylate cyclase second messenger system.

The PVN and medial prefrontal cortex were micropunch dissected from male Sprague-Dawley rats, pooled within brain regions and homogenized. Aliquots of a prepared membrane preparation were added to a reaction mixture consisting of 0.5 mM ATP, 2 mM $MgCl_2$, 0.5 mM IBMX, 0.7 mM HEPES, 0 or 10 uM GTP, 10 mM phosphocreatine, 5 U creatine phosphokinase and varying concentrations of CRF. Following a 20 min incubation at $30^{\circ}C$, the reaction was thermally ($95^{\circ}C$) terminated, the samples centrifuged (10,000g) and the cAMP content of the resulting supernatants determined by an automated radioimmunoassay (10). The results for 1 uM CRF, a maximally effective concentration for stimulating cAMP formation in responsive brain regions (7), are illustrated in Fig. 2. Consistent with previous reports (49,7), CRF produced a significant increase (166% of basal values) in cAMP formation in the medial prefrontal cortex. In contrast, CRF failed to alter cAMP formation in the PVN in the presence or absence of exogenous GTP. These results suggest that CRF receptors in the PVN, whether they reside on CRF or non-CRF-containing cells, are not coupled to adenylate cyclase-catalyzed cAMP synthesis. Therefore, the biochemical and molecular mechanisms involved in the transduction of CRF receptor occupancy in the PVN differ from that of other receptor populations in the CNS and are currently unknown.

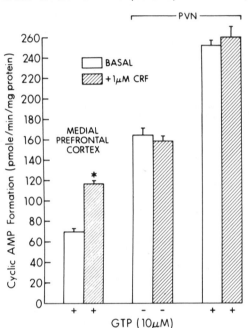

FIG 2. Effect of CRF and GTP on
adenylate cyclase activity in
homogenates of the paraventricular
nucleus of the hypothalamus (PVN)
and medial prefrontal cortex of the
rat.

CURRENT APPROACHES TO THE QUANTITATIVE RADIOIMMUNOASSAY
OF CIRCULATING ACTH

Any study of the HPA axis faces the immediate problem of
accurately assessing the functional output of the various components of
the axis. Most often, this is accomplished using radioimmunoassay
techniques (RIA). Most endocrine laboratories, using commercially
available RIAs, are capable of quantitating the common pituitary
hormones and adrenal steroids. When one examines these RIAs carefully,
however, they are often found lacking in requisite accuracy and
precision which limits their application. This is especially true when
one attempts to assess basal, particularly pulsatile, circulating levels
of these analytes. The low circulating concentrations, structural
homology with other products of post translational processing, and short
plasma half lives of these hormones and steroids all contribute to the
technical problems involved in their precise quantification. Recently,

with the advent of improved RIA techniques, procedures have become available which can accurately quantitate these analytes under basal conditions. The quantification of plasma Adrenal Corticotrophic Hormone (ACTH) exemplifies some of the problems inherent in assessing HPA axis functionality.

ACTH is a peptide composed of 39 amino acids and is derived from the post-translational processing of proopiomelanocortin (POMC) in the human anterior pituitary. The fact that ACTH is derived from a large precursor molecule which can be processed to yield a variety of distinct peptides has led to problems in producing antibodies specific for ACTH relative to other POMC products. The biological activity (i.e. steroidogenic activity) of the ACTH molecule appears to reside in the 1 – 20 amino acid subsequence of the molecule, and the 1 – 13 subsequence of ACTH is identical with that of alpha Melanocyte Stimulating Hormone (αMSH). Issues concerning the production of specific antibodies to ACTH have been dealt with in other reviews (40) and will not be discussed in detail here. Suffice it to say that any antisera used to quantitate plasma ACTH should be thoroughly characterized for cross reacting fragments and peptides. Ideally, the epitope of the antibody should be directed against some portion of the 1 –24 subsequence of the peptide in order to maximize the correlation of immunoreactivity (IR) with bioactivity and minimize cross-reactivity with αMSH.

Once a suitably specific antibody or antiserum has been obtained, several additional challenges remain in establishing an accurate and precise RIA of plasma ACTH (table 3). The lability of plasma ACTH has been verified by several workers (36,32) and thus the obtaining and processing of the sample is critical. The use of EDTA as an anticoagulant and a second centrifugation at 6,000 x G have been shown to slow the rate of disappearance of ACTH. Also, the use of peptidase inhibitors (i.e. Trasylol, 500 KIU/ml) have been shown to be effective in preserving ACTH in plasma. Care must be taken in choosing the concentration of peptidase inhibitor and anticoagulant as both have been shown to interfere with antigen-antibody binding at concentrations greater than 1 mM. Alternatively, acidification (pH ca. 2.0) of plasma supernatants also retards the degradation of ACTH. The whole blood and plasma are of course maintained at 4°C at all times during their processing. Also, since ACTH readily adsorbs to glass surfaces, both plastic tubes and pipette tips are used exclusively during the processing of samples.

The lability of solutions of authentic ACTH standards and radioiodinated ACTH is similar to that demonstrated for other peptide hormones. The preparation of stable ACTH solutions at concentrations less than 1 ug/ml requires the addition of trace amounts of albumin or poly-1-lysine and reduction of pH to < 3.5.

The low basal levels of circulating ACTH in man represent values which approach the limits of detection of many RIA techniques. A usable RIA for quantifying plasma ACTH should have an ED_{50} of approximately 100 pg/ml and a working limit of detection (two standard deviations greater than blank values) of 1 pg/ml. To attain these goals most ACTH RIAs utilize saturation binding kinetics (i.e. delayed trace addition) and second antibody separation technology. Additionally, the specific

Table 3

CHALLENGES INHERENT TO DETERMINATIONS OF CIRCULATING CONCENTRATIONS OF ACTH

1)	Short plasma half-life (rapid degradation in plasma)	approx. 5 to 7 minutes
2)	Low circulating concentrations	< 5 pg/ml (at times)
3)	Complex nature of plasma matrix	Other (non-ACTH) plasma proteins often interfere with antigen-antibody binding
4)	standard solutions	unstable below 1 ug/ml unless add albumin and reduce pH
5)	^{125}I-trace	not stable for more then 30 days

activity of monoiodinated (^{125}I) ACTH (ca. 400 uCi/ug), typically results in the use of low levels of tracer, usually between 2000 and 4000 cpm per assay tube. These factors taken in combination necessitate both precise pipetting and accurate radioactivity counting.

The direct quantification of ACTH in unextracted plasma by RIA has been hindered by the strong inhibition of binding exhibited by plasma components. To circumvent this problem, various liquid-liquid and liquid-solid extraction techniques were developed, including acid-acetone-ether extractions, the use of silicic acid (17), extraction with QUSO glass (8), and extraction on VYCOR glass powder (22). All of these methods are based on the adsorption of ACTH to silicates and its subsequent elution with acetic acid or acetic acid-acetone. The above methods are cumbersome, time consuming, and severely limit the number of samples which can be processed daily. In 1984, Nicholson and coworkers published the first practical RIA for the quantification of ACTH in unextracted human plasma. The development of the unextracted ACTH RIA was made possible by a more thorough understanding of the role of the sample matrix in RIA determinations. Nicholson and his colleagues observed the inappropriately high levels of ACTH in unextracted plasma and in plasma which had been "stripped" of ACTH. When diluted, this "immunoreactive ACTH" from stripped plasma consistently produced curves that were not parallel with standard curves generated using authentic ACTH. Using gel filtration, the "immunoreactive ACTH" content of stripped plasma appeared to be associated with higher molecular weight plasma proteins. This immunoreactivity did not represent either native hormone in some altered form or ACTH tracer binding to plasma proteins and co-eluted with bovine serum albumin (BSA) on a G-50 Sephadex column. Since this interference seems to reside in the large molecular weight fraction of plasma a viable strategy was to attempt to "blank out" this interference by saturating the sites of non-specific interaction with similar large molecular weight molecules. This approach is like that used in many commercial prolactin assays where cross-reactivity with human growth hormone is a problem. To this end, Nicholson and coworkers reported that a solution of 35 g BSA/liter closely mimicked the confounding effect observed in stripped plasma. This strategy must be used cautiously to avoid "blanking out" the antigen-antibody binding of interest. Ideally, the blanking agent used will be specific for the non-specific sites of interaction. Also, plasma samples may vary greatly in the amount of the interfering substance they contain. Unless dilution curves are run on every sample and parallelism with the standard curve is established it remains uncertain if all of the interfering sites have been "blanked out". Even the authors who proposed this strategy (8) state "when we use this method, most unextracted plasma specimens generated parallel competitive-binding curves, and their calculated plasma ACTH concentrations correlated well with those determined by a more laborious RIA of silicic acid extracts of the same plasma specimens", and later "very occasional subjects' unextracted plasma still reproducibly generated non-parallel binding curves".

The concerns mentioned above do not negate the use of this technique but do require that it be used only by an enlightened investigator. As a result of the reports of Nicholson and coworkers several commercial RIAs have been introduced, purportedly capable of accurately quantifying basal ACTH levels in unextracted plasma. In 1985 we reported the results of a study (11) comparing our (Duke) ACTH RIA using extracted samples with that of the Vanderbilt group's and two commercially available unextracted RIAs. Those results are shown in Table 4. The results of the Duke and Vanderbilt assays were in excellent agreement while the two commercial assays consistently over-estimated the amount of ACTH present in the plasma.

Table 4

RIA OF PLASMA ACTH: INTERASSAY COMPARISON

PLASMA SAMPLE	DUKE	VANDERBILT	R.S.L.	I.N.C.
A	4	8	17	*
B	25	23	26	35
C	15	13	17	47
D	18	21	41	46
E	49	37	93	*
F	32	38	51	757
G	8	10	39	*

Values represent pg ACTH/ml plasma

* not assayed

The use of alkyl bonded microparticulate silica (e.g. C_{18}) has been demonstrated to be a useful alternative to silicates as a means of prepurifying samples by solid phase extraction. The extraction is rapid (one person can easily extract 100 samples in a single working day) and efficient (recovery generally exceeds 85%). If ACTH standard curves are prepared in stripped plasma and processed by the same extraction technique no correction for recovery loss is necessary.

Figure 3 provides a step-wise description of a solid phase extracted ACTH RIA developed in our laboratory. The procedure is relatively straight forward, highly reproducible and satisfies the requirements for the assay of basal concentrations of circulating ACTH. Additionally, the solid phase extracts can also be used to quantitate circulating β-endorphin and arg-8-vasopressin. It should be stressed that both approaches (solid phase extraction or interference blanking) are valid strategies for quantifying basal levels of circulating ACTH. Both require vigilance by the investigator in order to insure accurate and precise results.

Recently, two interesting procedures have been published which seek to improve the assay of plasma ACTH measurements by incorporating immunoradiometric (IRMA) assay technology. In the first of these procedures (23) the authors used two epitope-distinct antibodies, one directed at the amino terminus and one directed against the carboxyl terminus of ACTH. The carboxy-terminus-directed antibody was coupled to CnBr-Sepharose and the amino-terminus-directed antibody was iodinated with ^{125}I to a high specific activity. Assay specificity is thus improved as a potential interferent would have to appreciably interact with both the first and second antibodies to pose a problem. In the second assay procedure (16) the authors utilize the same IRMA technology but label their detection antibody with a fluorometric rather than a radioactive tag. According to the authors, this assay is as precise and sensitive as any available RIA and has the additional benefit of a non-isotopic label which is stable for at least 50 weeks.

In summary we have enumerated, using ACTH as an example, the analytical and methodological considerations inherent in the accurate, precise and reproducible quantification of circulating pituitary hormones. In many ways our knowledge of the function of this hormone has paralleled the development of quantitative RIA technologies. It is tempting to speculate that our understanding of the neuroendocrine functions of the hypothalamus will soon parallel that of the pituitary as techniques are developed to measure in situ the dynamics and regulation of releasing factors produced there. There is however a point where the structural similarity between compounds becomes so great that even RIA technology is incapable of accurate measurement. This is exemplified by the steroids produced in the adrenal gland. Currently only GC/MS technology offers sufficient promise to accurately measure all the active steroids produced by this gland. In the next section we shall discuss the use of this powerful assay technique to further our understanding of HPA activity.

THE BIOHANDLING OF DEXAMETHASONE IN DEPRESSIVE DISORDERS: APPLICATION OF GAS CHROMATOGRAPHY/MASS SPECTROMETRY (GC/MS)

The Dexamethasone Suppression Test (DST) represents the most extensively applied of a group of provocative neuroendocrine challenge tests for the study and diagnosis of depression (12). Typically, a

Figure 3

FLOW DIAGRAM OF DUKE CLINICAL PSYCHOBIOLOGY LABORATORY RIA FOR PLASMA ACTH

Sample collection

1. Obtain blood sample in pre-chilled EDTA tube
2. Centrifuge specimen ($2-4^{o}C$, 2000g, 10 min)
3. Separate plasma, acidify (0.2ml 1M HCl/ml plasma)
4. Freeze immediately and transfer to laboratory
5. Recentrifuge sample ($2^{o}C$, 6000g, 10 min)

Sample preparation

1. Sep-Pak^{R} extraction

    a. Rinse
       i.   methanol
       ii. 8M urea
       iii. deionized H_2O

    b. Sample application (up to 40 ml plasma)

    c. Wash
       i. deionized H_2O
       ii. 4% acetic acid

    d. Elute with 4% acetic acid in 90% ethanol
       (fraction contains ACTH, β-endorphin and vasopressin)

2. Concentrate Sep-Pak extracts on rotary lyophilizer

3. Resuspend extract in 0.1% human serum albumin in H_2O, pH 3.60

ACTH RIA

1. 250 ul of solubilized ACTH extract
2. 100 ul 1/80,000 ACTH antibody 21-7
3. Incubate 18 to 24 hrs. at $4^{o}C$
4. 100 ul ^{125}I-ACTH (ca. 5,000 cpm), incubate 5 hrs. at $4^{o}C$
5. 20 ul second antibody, incubate 1 hr. at $4^{o}C$
6. 2ml deionized H_2O, centrifuge (2500g, 20 min, $4^{o}C$)
7. Decant tubes and count pellets

standardized dose of dexamethasone (e.g. 1 mg) is administered at 2300 hr and blood samples are obtained at 0800 and/or 1700 hr on the following day for determination of cortisol concentration. Subjects are distinguished based upon the suppression or early escape (nonsuppression) of cortisol secretion by dexamethasone, by reference to a predefined cut-off criterion (e.g. 5 ug cortisol/dl). Recent studies have suggested that the distinction between suppressors and nonsuppressors may be mediated, at least in part, by group differences in dexamethasone pharmacokinetics. Results of these studies indicate that nonsuppressors have significantly lower circulating concentrations of dexamethasone compared to suppressors and that blood dexamethasone concentrations are inversely correlated to post-DST cortisol values

(26,4,38,28). It should be emphasized that several studies have not demonstrated any significant differences in post–DST plasma dexamethasone concentration between suppressors and non–suppressors (13,46). However, all of these studies have several points in common including the exclusive use of RIA techniques for quantitating serum or plasma dexamethasone and the observation of a remarkably wide range of observed dexamethasone concentrations in both patient and control groups at standardized times following dexamethasone administration. The possibility certainly exists that the values obtained by RIA are contaminated due to cross–reactivity of the antibody with bioformed metabolites of dexamethasone, the identities of which have not been elucidated. Consistent with sound analytical practice, the results obtained by RIA must be corroborated by a distinct assay procedure of proven requisite sensitivity and specificity prior to speculating as to the significance of the aforementioned results.

In collaboration with Dr. James Vrbanac of the CLINSPEC program at the Medical School of South Carolina we have sought to develop a GC/MS assay for plasma dexamethasone using stable isotopically labelled dexamethasone as an internal standard. The monitoring of selected ions corresponding to generated fragments of a derivative of dexamethasone following its separation by capillary gas chromatography (mass fragmentography) offers distinct advantages over RIA techniques in terms of assay specificity while having comparable sensitivity. A mass fragmentographic assay for dexamethasone has been previously described (29) though has not been applied to the question of differences in the pharmacokinetics of dexamethasone in DST suppressors vs. nonsuppressors. The following discussion describes our current and developing techniques of sample preparation, derivatization, separation and detection for the mass fragmentographic assay of plasma dexamethasone.

Following the addition of 2 or 5 ng of [1,2,3,4,10,19-$^{13}C_6$,19,19,19-$^2H_3$]dexamethasone (a generous gift from Dr. James Freeman, Jefferson, Arkansas), plasma samples are prepurified either by Sep-Pak^R extraction or by immunoaffinity chromatography. The cartridge or column eluates are evaporated to dryness under nitrogen or lyophilized and the residue is reacted with 20 ul of a solution of 100 ug methoxylamine HCl/ul dry pyridine for 4 hrs at $60°C$. The mixture is subsequently evaporated to dryness under nitrogen and the product is solubilized in distilled water and extracted into ethyl acetate. Following evaporation of the solvent, 20 ul of N,O-bis(Trimethylsilyl) trifluoroacetamide (BSTFA) with 1% trimethylchlorosilane is added and the mixture heated for 1 hr at $80°C$. The resulting 3,20–dimethoxime–21–trimethylsilyl (diMO–TMS) derivative is injected onto a 2 m Ultra–1 fused silica capillary column (0.2 mm, i.d.) (Hewlett–Packard) and chromatographed by temperature programming the column oven (retention time of 4.9 min). The operating parameters for the mass spectrometer (Hewlett–Packard 5970B) were 70 eV for the electron energy, 2400V for the electron multiplier and the ion current at m/z 491 (nonlabelled dexamethasone) and m/z 500 (labelled dexamethasone) are monitored. The limit of assay detection defined by a signal–to–noise ratio of 5:1 is 100 pg and calibration curves generated by the addition of varying amounts of dexamethasone to plasma aliquots are linear to at least 20 ng/ml.

The mass spectrum of diMO–TMS derivatives of dexamethasone and $^{13}C_6$–$^2H_3$–dexamethasone is characterized by a parent ion at m/z 522 (531), a monitored ion at m/z 491 (500) of high relative abundance and a base peak at m/z 432 (441) (Figure 4). No evidence of the protium form of dexamethasone is observed in total ion chromatograms of diMO–TMS derivatives of $^{13}C_6$–$^2H_3$–dexamethasone. The diMO–TMS derivative of dexamethasone exhibits excellent GC properties, electron impact ionization efficiency and can be reproducibly and quantitatively formed. Attempts to additionally derivatize the sterically hindered hydroxyl groups in positions 11 and 17 were hindered by their unreliable formation and the use of reaction conditions and reagents which significantly prolonged assay time and necessitated the use of extensive clean–up of the reaction products. Mass chromatograms resulting from the selected ion monitoring of m/z 491 and 500 of diMO–TMS derivations of Sep–Pak^R extracts of 1ml of plasma to which 2ng of dexamethasone and $^{13}C_6$–$^2H_3$–dexamethasone were added are shown in Figure 5. Additional assay specificity may be obtained by monitoring the current ratio for an additional ion pair (i.e. 432/441) due to the high relative absorbance of this fragment.

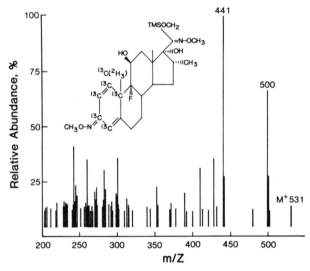

FIG 4. Partial mass spectrum of diMO–TMS derivative of $^{13}C_6$–$^3H_3$–dexamethasone.

In summary, we have attempted in this discussion to illustrate anatomical, biochemical and analytical approaches to the study of the functional organization and regulation of the HPA axis. In concert with molecular and cellular techniques, these approaches represent valuable avenues of preclinical and clinical research seeking to define the physiology and pathophysiology of the HPA axis.

Acknowledgements

This work was supported by a grant from the National Institutes of Mental health (MH39967) and the CLINSPEC program of the National Institutes of Health. The authors gratefully acknowledge the efforts of

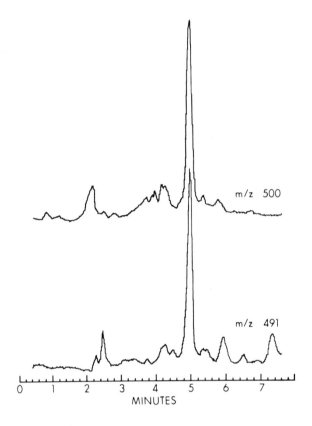

FIG 5. Mass fragmentograms of diMO-
TMS derivatives of dexamethasone
(m/z 491) and $^{13}C_6-^{3}H_3$-dexamethasone
(m/z 500) extracted from plasma.

Carl Anderson and Dr. Garth Bissette in these endeavors and the
assistance of Gail Atwater in the preparation of this manuscript.

References

1.   Agnati, L.F., Fuxe, K., Yu, Z.-Y., Harfstrand, A., Okret, S.,
     Wikstrom, A.-C., Goldstein, M., Zoli, M., Vale, W., and
     Gustafsson, J.-A. (1985): *Neurosci. Lett.*, 54:147-152.

2.   Aguilera, G., Harwood, J.P., Wilson, J.X., Morell, J., Brown,
     J.H., and Catt, K.J. (1983): *J. Biol. Chem.*, 258:8039-8045.

3.   Aguilera, G., Wynn, P.C., Harwood, J.P., Hauger, R.L., Millan,
     M.A., Grewe, C., and Catt, K.J. (1986): *Prog. Neuroendocrinol.*,
     43:79-88.

4. Arana, G.W., Workman, R.J., and Baldessarini, R.J. (1984): *Am. J. Psychiat.*, 141:1619–1621.

5. Axelrod, J. (1962): *J. Biol. Chem.*, 237:1657–1660.

6. Axelrod, J., and Reisine, T. (1984): *Science*, 224:452–459.

7. Battaglia, G., Webster, E., and DeSouza, E.B. (1987): *Mol. Pharmacol.*, in press.

8. Berson, A.A. and Yallow, R.S. (1968): *J. Clin. Invest.*, 47:2725–2749.

9. Besser, G.M., Orth, D.N., Nicholson, W.E., Byyny, R.L., Abe, K., and Woodham, J.P. (1971): *J. Clin. Endocrinol.*, 32:595–603.

10. Brooker, G., Harper, J.F., Teraski, W.L., and Moylan, R.D. (1979): In: *Advances in Cyclic Nucleotide Reserach*, Vol. 10, edited by G. Brooker, P. Greengard, and G.A. Robison, pp. 1–32, Raven Press, New York.

11. Bruhn, T.O., Plotsky, P.M., and Vale, V.W. (1984): *Endocrinol.*, 114:57–62.

12. Carroll, B.J., Feinberg, M., Greden, J.F., Tarika, J., Albaala, A.A., Haskett, R.J., James, N.M., Kronfol, Z., Lohr, N., Steiner, M., de Vigne, J.P., and Young, E. (1981): *Arch. Gen. Psychiat.*, 38:15–22.

13. Carroll, B.J., Schroeder, K., Mukhopadhyay, S., Greden, J.R., Feinberg, M., Ritchie, J., and Tarika, J. (1980): *J. Clin. Endocrinol. Metab.*, 51:433–437.

14. Chappell, P.B., Smith, M.A., Kilts, C.D., Bissette, G., Ritchie, J., Anderson, C., and Nemeroff, C.B. (1986): *J. Neurosci.*, 6:2908–2914.

15. De Souza, E.B., Insel, T.R., Perrin, M.H., Rivier, J., Vale, W.V., and Kuhar, M.J. (1985): *J. Neurosci.*, 5:3189–3203.

16. Dobson, S., White, A., Hoadley, M., Jougren, T., and Ratcliffe, J. (1987): *Clin. Chem.*, in press.

17. Donald, R.A. (1967): *Endocrinol.*, 39:451–452.

18. Feldman, S. (1985): *Fed. Proc.*, 44:169–176.

19. Fuller, R.W., Hemrick-Luecke, S., Toomey, R.E., Horng, J.-S., Ruffolo, R.R., Jr., and Molloy, B.B. (1981): *Biochem. Pharmacol.* 30:1345–1352.

20. Ganong, W.F. (1980): *Fed. Proc.*, 39:2923.

21. Giguere, V., Labrie, F., Cote, J., and Coy, D.H. (1982): *Proc. Nat. Acat. Sci. USA*, 79:3466–3469.

22. Gutkowska, J., Julesz, J., St.-Louis, J., and Genest, J. (1982): *Clin. Chem.*, 28:2229–2234.

23. Hodgkinson, S.C., Allolio, B., Landon, J., and Lowry, P.J. (1984): *Biochem. J.*, 218:703–711.

24. Hokfelt, Johansson, O., and Goldstein, M. (1984): In: *Handbook of Chemical Neuroanatomy. Classical Neurotransmitters in the CNS Part I.*, edited by A. Bjorklund and T. Hokfelt, pp. 157–276. Elsevier, New York.

25. Hollt, V. and Haarman, I. (1984): *Biochem. Biophys. Res. Comm.*, 124:407–415.

26. Holsboer, F., Haak, D., Gerken, A., and Vecsei, P. (1984): *Biol. Psychiat.*, 19:281–291.

27. Isaacson, R.L. (1982): *The Limbic System*. Plenum Press, New York.

28. Johnson, G.F., Hunt, G., Kerr, K., Caterson, I. (1984): *Psychiat. Res.*, 13:305–313.

29. Kasuya, Y., Althaus, J.R., Freeman, J.P., Mitchum, R.K., and Skelly, J.P. (1982): *J. Pharmaceut. Sci.*, 73:446–451.

30. Kilts, C.D. and Anderson, C.M. (1986): *Neurochem. Int.*, 9:437–445.

31. Kilts, C.D. and Anderson, C.M. (1987): *Brain Res.*, in press.

32. Lambert, A., Frost, J., Ratcliff, W.A., and Robertson, W.R. (1985): *Clin. Endocrinol.*, 253–261:1344.

33. Liposits, Zs., Paull, W.K., Setalo, G., and Vigh, S. (1985): *Histochem.*, 83:5–16.

34. Liposits, Zs, Phelix, C., and Paull, W.K. (1986): *Histochem.*, 84:201–205.

35. Makara, G.B., Stark, E., Karteszi, M., Palkovits, M., and Rappay, G. (1981): *Am. J. Physiol.*, 240:E441–E446.

36. Matsuyama, H., Ruhmann-Wenhold, A., Johnson, L.R., and Nelson, D.H. (1972): *Metabolism*, 21:30–35.

37. Mezey, E., Kiss, J.Z., Skirboll, L.R., Goldstein, M., and Axelrod, J. (1984): *Nature*, 310:140–141.

38. Morris, H., Carr, V., Gilliland, J., and Hooper, M. (1986): *Br. J. Psychiat.*, 148:66–69.

39. Nicholson, W.E., Davis, D.R., Sherrell, B.J., and Orth, D.N. (1984): *Clin. Chem.*, 30:259–265.

40. Orth, D.N. (1979): In: *Methods of Hormone Radioimmunoassay*, edited by B.M. Jaffe, H.R. Behrman, 2nd ed., pp. 245-284, Academic Press, New York.

41. Palkovits, M. (1973): *Brain Res.*, 59:449-450.

42. Palkovits, M. (1975): *Anatom. Neuroendocrinol.*, 72-80.

43. Palkovits, M., Brownstein, M., Saavedra, J.M., and Axelrod, J. (1974): *Brain Res.*, 77:137-149.

44. Reisine, T., Affolter, H.-U., Rougon, G., and Barbet, J. (1986): *TINS*, Nov./Dec.

45. Ritchie, J.C., Kegelmeyer, A.E., and Walker, J.T. (1985): *Soc. for Neurosci. Abstr.*

46. Rubin, R.T, Poland, R.E., Blodgert, A.L.N., Winston, R.A., Forster, B., and Carroll, B.J. (1980): In: *Progress in Psychoneuroendocrinology*, edited by F. Brambilla, G. Racagni, and D. de Weids, pp. 223-234, Elsevier/North Holland Biomedical Press, New York.

47. Smythe, G.A. Bradshaw, J.E., and Vining, R.F. (1983): *Endocrinol.*, 113:1062-1071.

48. Swanson, L.W., Sawchenko, P.I., Rivier, J., and Vale, W.V. (1983): *Neuroendocrinol.*, 36:165-186.

49. Wynn, P.C., Hauger, R.L., Holmes, M.C., Millan, M.A., Catt, K.J., and Aguilera, G. (1984): *Peptides*, 5:1077-1084.

The Hypothalamic-Pituitary-Adrenal Axis:
Physiology, Pathophysiology, and Psychiatric
Implications, edited by A.F. Schatzberg and
C.B. Nemeroff. Raven Press, Ltd., New York
© 1988.

BEHAVIORAL EFFECTS OF CORTICOTROPIN

RELEASING FACTOR

Karen Thatcher Britton and George F. Koob*

Department of Psychiatry, Veterans Administration Medical Center and
UCSD School of Medicine, La Jolla, CA 92161

*Division of Preclinical Neuroscience and Endocrinology, Scripps Clinic
10666 North Torrey Pines Road, La Jolla, CA 92037

A convergence of evidence suggests that changes in the functional
activity of the hypothalamic–pituitary–adrenal (HPA) axis and
sympathetic nervous system may be important in the pathophysiology of
stress, anxiety and depression. Many patients with primary depressive
illness have high cerebrospinal fluid CRF levels (Nemeroff, 1984) as
well as elevated cortisol production, alterations in normal cortisol
periodicity, and an abnormal dexamethasone suppression test (Carroll et
al, 1976). Similar evidence of HPA hyperactivity has been reported in
patients with alcoholism (Stokes, 1973), anorexia nervosa (Gerner and
Gwirtzman, 1981), bulimia (Gwirtzman et al, 1983), obsessive–compulsive
disorder (Insel et al, 1982), and dementia (Spar and Gerner, 1982).
Patients with adrenocortical hyperactivity and deficiencies states also
have been reported to show a range of psychiatric disturbances as have
patients receiving large doses of adrenocortical and synthetic steroids
(Ling et al, 1981). However, identification of the possible brain
mechanisms which could participate in influencing these neurobehavioral
changes have not been elucidated.

The sequencing and subsequent synthesis of corticotropin releasing
factor (CRF) (Vale et al, 1981) has provided a direct opportunity to
study the central control of the HPA axis, and numerous studies support
the hypothesis that CRF is the critical mediator of stress–induced
changes in the pituitary adrenocortical response to stress. Although
CRF was originally isolated and characterized on the basis of its
ability to induce ACTH release, it is now known to exert a surprisingly
broad spectrum of action. CRF appears to act within the brain as a
mediator of certain autonomic nervous system, visceral and behavioral
actions independent of its action on the pituitary. These effects are
not abolished by extirpation of the anterior pituitary or by removal of
the target endocrine glands. These actions, in concert with the wide
anatomical distribution of CRF in brain regions outside the areas

involved in the regulation of anterior pituitary function (Swanson et al, 1983), provide a tenable basis for hypothesizing that CRF may simultaneously activate and coordinate neuroendocrine, autonomic, circulatory, metabolic and behavioral responses to stressful stimuli.

In support of this hypothesis are the findings that CRF has central nervous system activating properties at the cellular (Aldenhoff et al, 1982), electroencephalographic (Ehlers et al, 1983) and behavioral (Sutton et al, 1982) level when administered directly into the central nervous system. Intracerebral injection of CRF produces elevation of plasma epinephrine, norepinephrine and glucose (Brown et al, 1982; Brown and Fisher, 1983). These effects are reproduceable in hypophysectomized, adrenalectomized animals, but abolished by ganglionic blocking agents (Brown and Fisher, 1983). Intraventricular injections of CRF also produce a profound dose-dependent activation of the EEG (Ehlers et al, 1983). At a more cellular level CRF has been shown to produce a pronounced depolarization and excitation of hippocampal and other neurons (Aldenhoff et al, 1982) Furthermore, CRF produced increases in the firing frequencies of cells within the locus coeruleus (Valentino et al, 1983), a system thought to be of importance in the mechanism by which the brain is able to attend selectively to certain novel external events (Foote et al, 1983).

Role of CRF in Behavior

The hypothesis that CRF also might be involved in the regulation of behavioral responsiveness was based on two considerations. First, the neuroanatomical distribution of CRF in extensive extra-hypothalamic sites in the spinal cord, brainstem, and diencephalic regions of the central nervous system (Olshowka, et al, 1982; Merchanthaler, 1984) could provide a morphological basis for CRF to act as a neurotransmitter or neuromodulator in ways analogous to more traditionally accepted neurotransmitters. Secondly, other hypophyseal (releasing and inhibiting) peptides have been shown to elicit behavioral actions, namely, thyrotropin releasing hormone (TRH), leutinizing hormone releasing hormone (LH-RH) and somatostatin (SS). These facts led to the original experiment which was designed to test the effect of CRF on general behavioral responsiveness.

Rats injected with icv CRF (15, 150 or 1500 picomoles) show a consistent and marked dose-dependent increase in activity as measured by photocell interruptions (Sutton et al, 1982). This increase in activity lasts for a period over five hours postinjection in the rats injected with 1500 picomoles of CRF. Besides normal locomotion and sniffing, the rats injected with CRF exhibit an interesting set of behaviors which appear to reflect a general behavioral activation. These behaviors include elevated walking, grooming and rearing Subcutaneous injections of CRF in doses as high as 7.5 nmoles failed to produce similar increases in locomotor activity in the photocell cages, suggesting that CRF is acting directly on the brain to produce behavioral activation.

In order to explore the contribution of the pituitary adrenal system to these behavioral effects, rats were pretreated with dexamethasone, a synthetic glucocorticoid that inhibits release of ACTH and corticosterone. Although dexamethasone effectively suppressed plasma corticosterone, it failed to alter or reverse icv CRF effects on locomotor activation (Britton et al, 1985), see Fig. 1. The behavioral

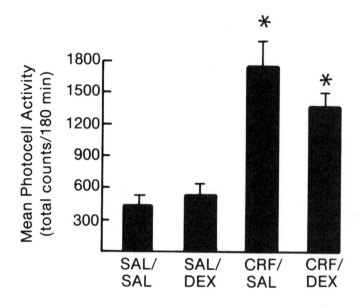

FIG 1. The interaction of CRF (1.0 μg, icv) and dexamethasone (100 μg/kg, i.p.) on locomotor activity in photocell cages. Results represent total activity counts over 3 hours (mean ± SEM). N=12 for saline and n=15 for other groups. * significantly different from saline treated group, p < .05.

activation by CRF can be further separated from the effects on the pituitary-adrenal system because hypophysectomized rats (chronically treated with rat growth hormone to control for weight) show equivalent increases in acivity after icv administration of CRF compared to sham-operated controls (Eaves et al, 1983) see Fig. 2. These results indicate that the pituitary-adrenal activity produced by central CRF administration is not a necessary condition for obtaining CRF-induced behavioral activation and provide further evidence for the hypothesis that CRF is acting at central sites within the CNS to produce these effects.

An important question is whether the behavioral effects of CRF are dependent on any classical neurotransmitter in the nervous system. The locomotor-activating properties of several stimulant compounds are believed to result from their ability to increase central dopamine transmission. Two approaches were used to evaluate whether dopamine plays a role in CRF-induced locomotor activation. First, rats previously treated with CRF (1 μg icv) were administered with ∝-flupenthixal, a dopamine receptor antagonist, and placed in photocell cages for monitoring locomotor activition. The CRF-induced locomotor activation was reversed by ∝-flupenthixal (i.p.); but only at doses

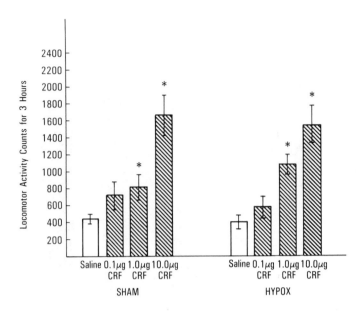

FIG 2. Effects of CRF on locomotor activity in photocell cages in hypophysectomized rats treated chronically with rat growth hormone and sham operated controls. Results represent the total activity counts over 3 hours (mean ± SEM). N=9 in each group. * significantly different from saline control, p < .05.

that cause catelepsy (Koob et al, 1984), see Fig. 3. Second, the locomotor activating properties of CRF were not blocked following 6-hydroxy dopamine lesions of the nucleus accumbens (Swerdlow and Koob, 1985). These results suggest that CRF acts independently of direct activation of dopamine transmission.

The opioid peptide system has also been implicated in mediating behavior activation. However, while naloxone antagonizes amphetamine-stimulated locomotion, it has no effect on CRF-induced behavioral activation (Koob et al, 1984). In fact, the only stimulatory compound studied that showed a similar pharmacological and behavioral profile to CRF was caffeine. Further studies are needed to ascertain whether caffeine and CRF might share some common neural substrate.

CRF and Stress

One of the earliest studies performed to ascertain whether CRF was a behaviorally active peptide was to expose a rat to a novel, open field environment and observe its behavior. Typically, a rat rejected icv with CRF shows a marked decrease in exploratory and ingestive behavior and remains close to the corners of the field, in contrast to an untreated animal which makes increasingly frequent forays into the center of the field to consume food (Britton et al, 1982; Sutton et al,

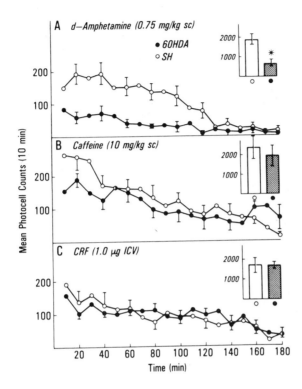

FIG 3. Locomotor response to (A) 0.75 mg/kg d-amphetamine, (B) 10 mg/kg caffeine and (C) 1.0 μg CRF in rats following sham (open circle) or 6-OHDA (darkened circle) lesions of the nucleus accumbens.

1982). These behaviors are consistent with heightened "emotionality" or increased sensitivity to the, presumably, stressful aspects of the test.

These findings led to the suggestion that CRF might be related in some way to the expression of human anxiety or fear. Since it is not possible to identify animals with anxiety, we chose to examine the effects of CRF in a series of tests that are animal models of anxiety or are sensitive to anxiolytic compounds.

One of the most consistent behavioral effects of antianxiety agents is their ability to "release" behavior previously suppressed by punishment, and one of the most sensitive animal models to measure this effect is the conflict test. The conflict test is an operant conditioning paradigm in which a reinforcing stimulus (food) is accompanied by an aversive stimulus (shock). Antianxiety agents consistently "release" or increase behaviors previously suppressed by punishment in the conflict test with a rank order of potency similar to that observed clinically (Cook and Sepinwall, 1975).

Rats treated with CRF display a pattern of responding in the conflict test that is the opposite to that observed in rats treated with benzodiazepines. CRF (0.5 and 1.0 μg, icv) produced a dose-dependent attenuation of both punished and non-punished responding on the conflict test, decreasing non-punished responding to 40% of baseline and the number of shocks taken to 55% of baseline (Figure 4). As expected, chlordiazepoxide (5 mg/kg i.p.) significantly increased the number of footshocks taken during the punishment component (not displayed). In addition, chlordiazepoxide reversed the response-attentuating effects of CRF, restoring non-punished responding to 75% of baseline and punished responding to nearly 100% of baseline, see Fig. 5. These results suggest that exogenously administerd CRF can produce changes in the rat consistent with an exaggeration of the stressfulness of the environment and that this behavioral state can be reversed by classical 'antianxiety' drugs.

Another paradigm differentially sensitive to anxiogenic and anxiolytic compounds is the acoustic startle test. The acoustic startle reflex is is an easily quantified muscular contraction in response to an intense acoustic stimulus. CRF (1 μg icv) significantly potentiates acoustic startle amplitude. Pretreatment with the benzodiazepine chlordiazepoxide in doses that do not by themselves lower startle baseline attenuates this effect. These results support the hypothesis that CRF might act to potentiate behavioral responses normally expressed during states of enhanced fear or anxiety.

Physiological role of CRF

When a naturally occurring neuropeptide is found to produce a specific behavioral effect, the question that arises is whether the effect is pharmacologically-induced or is it an effect that mimics a normally occurring state? The development of analogues specific antibodies and antagonists provides a tool for the study of the physiological influence that a peptide may exert on behavior.

For example, the physiological role of CRF in regulating ACTH release was originally demonstrated with passive immunization against CRF, which significantly reduced ACTH secretion in adrenalectomized rats and inhibited ether stress-induced rises in plasma ACTH in intact rats (Rivier et al, 1982). Similarly, a recently-developed CRF antagonist (α-helical CRF $_{9-41}$) suppresses ether-induced elevations of plasma epinephrine, but not norepineprine (Rivier et al, 1984; Brown et al 1984). Antisera to CRF have also been used for the detection of cell bodies and fibers containing the neuropeptide (Swanson et al, 1983).

We have begun preliminary behavioral testing utilizing a CRF antagonist(α-helical $_{9-41}$) in order to determine if the antagonist could reverse the behavioral effects of CRF in the conflict test and photocell activity cages. In addition, we were interested in ascertaining whether the antagonist possesses any intrinsic (possibly "anxiolytic-like") properties.

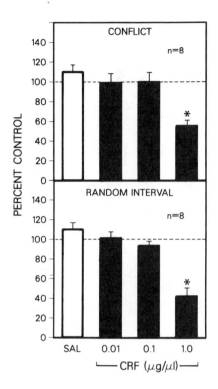

FIG 4. The effects of CRF on responding during the random interval (food alone on a RF 30-S schedule) and conflict (food and incremental shock delivered for each lever press) of an operant conflict test. * significantly different from saline control, P < .05.

Infusion of α-helical $_{9-41}$ (50,100 and 200 μg; icv, as a suspension)) attenuated CRF-induced locomotor activation as well as the response suppression observed in the conflict test, see Fig. 6. The antagonist appeared devoid of intrinsic activity in these particular behavioral tests. The ability of the CRF-A to block these effects suggests that an endogenous peptide is necessary for the naturally occurring expression of these behaviors.

Possible Clinical Relevance

Clearly, more information concerning physiological relevance of these findings is needed. The question of whether the CNS actions of the peptides are simply pharmacological or of physiological relevance is fundamental. The majority of the work on the CNS effects of CRF examines the effects of exogenous administrations. It is unknown at this time whether the endogenous neuropeptide actions are similar to those elicited by exogenous neuropeptide administration.

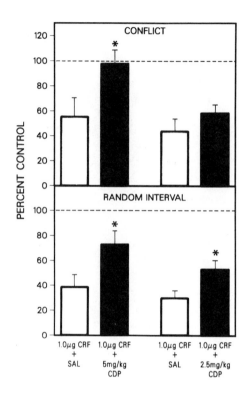

FIG 5. The interaction of CRF (1 µg icv) and
chlordiazepoxide on responding during the random
interval and conflict components of an operant
conflict test. * significantly different from CRF
alone, p < .05 main effect (CDP) ANOVA.

Considering the extensive literature linking CRF to stress, it is
not surprising that clinical studies have appeared suggesting that CRF
may play a role in mediating some forms of stress-related
psychopathology.   Cerebrospinal fluid levels of CRF are elevated in
many patients with depression (Nemeroff et al, 1984) and anorexia
nervosa (W. Kaye, Pers. Communic.). Abnormal activation of the HPA
axis has been reported in alcoholism (Stokes, 1973), bulemia (Gwirtzman
et al, 1983), and Alzheimer's Disease (Spar and Gerner, 1982) as well.

The hypothesis that stress may provoke or exacerbate clinical
depression has suggested for a number of years. Anisman and Zacharko
(1982) propose that stressful experiences engage behavioral and
neurochemical coping mechanisms. However, if behavioral control of the
stress is not achieved, neurochemical coping mechanisms cause depletion
of brain biogenic amines, producing affective disorders. In this
scheme, clinical depression is viewed as a maladaptive outcome of
partially successful attempts at adaptation. Central CRF stores may
also play an etiological role in depression in that the depressive

state may represent an oversuccessful adaptation ("overcompensation") to a hyperactive CRF system. However, the question of whether altered central stores of CRF might medate some of the behavioral aspects of depression remains to be elucidated.

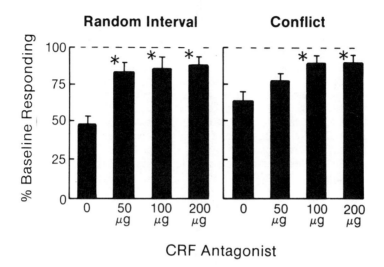

FIG 6. Effect of CRF receptor antagonist (50, 100 or 200 µg, icv) on CRF-induced (1.0 µg, icv) response suppression in the conflict test. * sigificantly different from controls, p < .05

PERSPECTIVE

Much of the current interest in CRF resides in the hypothesis that this neuropeptide plays an important role in the function of the brain independent of the pituitary gland. The experiments described herein support this hypotheis. What the central CRF receptors do, however, is far less clear.

For decades there has been speculation that the elusive CRF molecule might serve as the "first mediator of Stress-Responses" (Selye, 1956). While progress has been made in eliminating compounds such as adrenalin, noradrenalin, acetylcholine and histamine as not meeting the criteria for "first mediator", the issue of clarifying the substrates involved in the afferent limb of the stress response has been largely ignored.

On the other hand, numerous studies have emphasized the non-specificity of the pituitary-adrenal stress response to a variety of diverse stimuli. The efferent limb of the stress response appears nonspecific with respect to a variety of stimuli and is relatively slow to develop, especially in the periphery. This observation led Mason (1971) to hypothesize that the "primary mediator" underlying the pituitary adrenal response to various stressors may be the neural substrate for emotional arousal or alerting responses to threatening or aversive factors in general, i.e., a behavioral response preparatory to fight, flight or struggle in a threatening situation.

One might hypothesize that CRF may be not only the first mediator of the pituitary stress response but also may be involved in mobilizing the neural substrates for emotional arousal. Studies demonstrating that CRF elicits neuronal, sympathetic and behavioral activation, coupled with stress-enhancing actions that are responsive to anxiolytic compounds, suggest a posible role for corticotropin releasing factor in a fundamental activating system that mobilizes an organism to meet an environmental challenge. Questions such as what pathways project to CRF-secreting cells, what neurochemical changes are concerned with the regulation of CRF release and what are the interactions between central and pituitary-adrenal CRF systems remain to be elucidated.

REFERENCES

1. Anisman, H. and Zacharko, R. (1982): Behav. Brain Sci. 5:89–137.

2. Aldenhoff, J. B., Gurol, D. L. and Siggins, G. R. (1982): Neurosci. Abst. 8:983.

3. Britton, D. R., Koob, G. F., Rivier, J. and Vale W. (1982): Life Sci. 31:363–376.

4. Britton, K. T., Morgan, J., Rivier, J., Vale, W. and Koob, G. F. (1985): Psychopharmacology 86:170–174.

5. Britton, K. T., Lee, G., Dana. R., Risch, S. C. and Koob, G. F. (1986): Life Sci. 39:1281–1286.

6. Britton, K. T., Lee, G., Vale, W., Rivier, J. and Koob, G. F. (1986): Brain Res. 369:303–306.

7. Brown, M., Fisher, L., Rivier., J., Spiess, J., Rivier, C. and Vale, W. (1982): Life Sci. 30:207–210.

8. Brown, M. R. and Fisher, L. A. (1983): Brain Res. 280:75–79.

9. Brown, M. R., Fisher, L., Webb, V., Vale, W. and Rivier, J. (1985): Brain Res 328:355–357.

10. Carroll, B. J., Curtis, G. C. and Mendels, J. (1976): Arch. Gen. Psychiatry 33:1039–1058.

11. Cook, L., Sepinwall, J. (1975): In: Mechanism of Action of Benzodiazepines, edited by E. Costa and P. Greengard, pp. 1–28, Raven Press, New York.

12. Eaves, M. R., Britton, K. T., Rivier, J., Vale W. and Koob, G. (1985): Peptides 8:818–822.

13. Ehlers, C., Henriksen, S., Wang, M., Rivier, J., Vale, W. and Bloom, F. (1983): Brain Res. 278-332-336.

14. Foote, S., Bloom, F. E. and Aston-Jones, G. (1983): Physiol. Rev. Rev. 63:844–914.

15. Gerner, R. H. and Gwirtsman, H. E. (1981): Am. J. Psychiatry 138:650–653.

16. Gold, P. W., Gwirtsman, H., Averginus, P. C. et al. (1986): NEJM 314:1335–1342.

17. Gwirtsman, H. E., Roy-B¨rne, P., Yager, J., et al. (1983): Am. J. Psychiatry 140:559;563.

18. Insel, T. R., Kalin, W. H., Guttmacher, L. B., et al. (1982): Psychiatry Res. 6:153–160.

19, Koob, G. F., Swerdlow, N., Seeligson, M., Eaves, M., Sutton, R., Rivier, J. and Vale, W. (1984): Neuroendocrinology 39:459–464.

20. Ling, M., Perry, P. and Tsuang, M. (1981): Psychiatry 38:471–477.

21. Mason, J. W. (1971): J. Psychiat. Res. 8:323–333.

22. Merchenthaler, I. (1984): Peptides 5:53–69.

23. Nemeroff, C. B., Widerlove, E., Bissette, G., Walleus, H., Karlsson, I., Eklund, K., Kilts, C., Loosen, P. T. and Vale, W. (1984): Science 226:1342–1344.

24. Olschowka, J. A., O'Donohue, T. L., Mueller, G. P. and Jacobowitz, D. M. (1982): Neuroendocrinology 35:305–308.

25. Rivier, C., Rivier, J. and Vale, W. (1982): Science 218:377–379.

26. Rivier, J., Rivier, C. and Vale W. (1984): Science 224:889–891.

27. Selye, H. and Henser, G. (1956): In: Fifth Annual Report on Stress MD Publications, New York.

28. Spar, J. E. and Gerner, P. (1982): Amer. J. Psychiatry 139:238–240.

29. Stokes, P. E. (1973): An NY Acad. Sci. 215:77–84.

30: Sutton, R., Koob, G. F., LeMoal, M., Rivier, J. and Vale, W. (1982): Nature (London) 297-331-333.

31. Swanson, L., Sawcheko, P., Rivier, J. and Vale, W. (1983): Neuroendocrinology 36:165–186.

32. Swerdlow, N. and Koob, G. F. (1985): Pharmacol. Biochem. Behav. 23:303–307.

33. Swerdlow, N., Geyer, M. (1986): Psychopharmacology 88:147–152.

34. Vale, W., Spiess, J., Rivier, C. and Rivier, J. (1981): Science 213:1394–1397.

35. Valentino, R., Foot, S. and Aston-Jones, H. G. (1983): Brain Res. 270–363–367.

The Hypothalamic-Pituitary-Adrenal Axis:
Physiology, Pathophysiology, and Psychiatric
Implications, edited by A.F. Schatzberg and
C.B. Nemeroff. Raven Press, Ltd., New York
© 1988.

ALTERED HYPOTHALAMIC-PITUITARY-ADRENAL REGULATION

IN ANIMAL MODELS OF DEPRESSION

Ned H. Kalin and Lorey K. Takahashi

Psychiatry Service, William S. Middleton Memorial Veterans Hospital,
2500 Overlook Terrace, Madison, Wisconsin 53705
and
Department of Psychiatry, University of Wisconsin Medical School,
Madison, WI 53792

A prominent biological finding associated with depression is altered regulation of the hypothalamic-pituitary-adrenal (HPA) system. Traditionally, interest in neuroendocrine alterations associated with depression was based on the fact that brain neurotransmitter systems regulate endocrine function. To understand the pathophysiology of depression, it is also important to recognize that hormonal systems directly modulate neurotransmitter function and regulate motivational and behavioral systems. Intensive research efforts have been made to establish the mechanisms underlying the HPA dysregulation that occurs in depression. However, these studies are difficult and often impossible to perform in humans. Animal models of depression allow for in-depth mechanistic studies. In this chapter we review two prominent animal models of depression: attachment bond disruption in nonhuman primates and exposure to uncontrollable stress in rodents. These models were chosen because they produce behavioral changes analogous to human depression. In addition, separation and lack of control over stressors are important factors underlying human depression. The phenomenology and neurobiology of these animal models of depression will be examined in relation to the HPA system.

UNCONTROLLABLE STRESS AND LEARNED HELPLESSNESS

When animals are exposed to uncontrollable stressful situations, alterations in behavior commonly referred to as learned helplessness are produced. The learned helplessness phenomenon was first described by Seligman and colleagues (33,39). They reported that dogs exposed to yoked inescapable electric shocks showed severe deficits in subsequent performance in situations where escape from aversive stimuli was possible. In marked contrast, dogs exposed to the same shock schedules but given behavioral control over the termination of shock later exhibited adaptive escape responses when exposed to noxious stimuli. Thus, lack of control over a stressor facilitates the onset and subsequent manifestation of learned helplessness.

Since these initial experiments, considerable research has been directed toward uncovering the physiological bases of learned helplessness and other consequences of exposure to uncontrollable stress. For example, studies using neurochemical techniques have revealed that exposure to uncontrollable, but not controllable, shock results in a significant reduction in brain concentrations of norepinephrine (1,52). Consistent with these findings, pharmacological enhancement of norepinephrine and dopamine levels blocks the behavioral effects of uncontrollable shock (2). Taken together, these findings suggest that depletion of brain catecholamines may underlie the behavioral depression induced by uncontrollable stress. Exposure to uncontrollable stress results in additional physiological changes, including decreased sensitivity to nociceptive stimuli (14) and reduced immune system responsiveness (25).

In contrast to the numerous neurochemical and neuropharmacological reports, fewer studies have examined the consequences of both uncontrollable and controllable stressors on the regulation of HPA hormones. We focus this section on studies directly comparing the effects of controllable stressors with those of uncontrollable stressors on HPA activation. Studies that only compare the effects of uncontrollable stress with those of no stress are unable to distinguish the effects of uncontrollability from the effects of the stressor.

To unravel the contribution of HPA hormones in mediating the effects of controllable and uncontrollable stressors, researchers have utilized two major strategies. One strategy is to determine the hormonal profile of the animal after confronting an uncontrollable or controllable stressor. Typically, animals are killed at a predetermined time after the treatment and blood levels of various hormones are assayed. Another strategy is to remove endocrine glands and administer hormones exogenously to establish the role of a specific hormone in mediating behavioral depression.

Pituitary Adrenocorticotropic Hormone (ACTH)

In the only published study that has examined the effects of controllable and uncontrollable stressors on ACTH release, Maier et al. (30) reported that rats showed elevated ACTH levels after exposure to one session of escapable or yoked inescapable electric tail-shocks. The elevated ACTH levels declined gradually and approached baseline levels 24 h after shock treatment. However, ACTH values did not differ significantly between the two groups.

Because one session of uncontrollable shock did not produce higher ACTH levels than controllable shock, we investigated the effects of repeated treatment with escapable and inescapable shock on ACTH release. Male rats were exposed to escapable or yoked inescapable tail-shocks every three days for nine sessions of 80 shocks in wheel-turn boxes identical to those used in the study by Maier et al. (30). Control rats were restrained in the apparatus but did not receive shocks. Seventy-two hours after the last stress session, one half of the rats in the escapable and inescapable shock groups were decapitated and plasma was collected for hormonal analysis. Control rats were also decapitated at this time. The remaining animals were tested again in their respective condition and killed promptly after exposure to 20 shocks. The results indicated that ACTH levels did not differ significantly 72 h after the ninth session of controllable or uncontrollable shock treatment. However, the additional exposure to 20 shocks significantly enhanced ACTH concentrations in rats that had been repeatedly exposed to uncontrollable shock (Fig. 1). This is the first demonstration of differential regulation of ACTH secretion occurring after chronic uncontrollable stress treatments. Further research is needed to determine whether the enhanced release of ACTH occurs in other stressful situations after chronic exposure to uncontrollable stress.

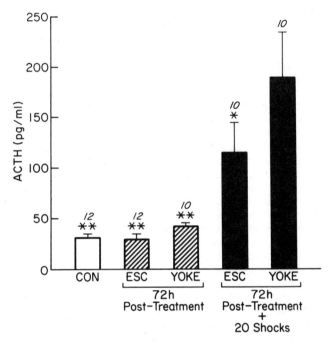

FIG. 1. Plasma ACTH levels after repeated exposure to escapable (ESC), yoked inescapable (YOKE), or no shock (CON) treatment. The SEM and number of animals are shown above each bar. * p < .05, ** p < .01 (significantly different from the yoked group that was given 20 shocks).

No studies have specifically assessed the role of ACTH in mediating the learned helplessness response. Manipulations such as hypophysectomy and dexamethasone treatment have been performed, but they reduce both ACTH and corticosterone. Furthermore, neither hypophysectomy nor dexamethasone treatment eliminates the motivational deficits associated with uncontrollable stress exposure (28).

Glucocorticoids

Numerous studies have examined the immediate poststress effects produced by controllable and uncontrollable shock on glucocorticoid levels. For example, Weiss (50,51) reported that both controllable and uncontrollable tail-shock produced similar increases in corticosterone levels that were significantly higher than after no shock. These findings have been confirmed by other investigators (30,46,49).

Studies have also examined the changes in corticosterone levels over time in animals exposed to escapable or inescapable stress. Swenson and

Vogel (45) and Maier et al. (30) reported elevated corticosterone levels in both escapable and inescapable conditions immediately after stress treatments. However, Swenson and Vogel reported that animals in the inescapable stress group continued to exhibit elevated corticosterone values for up to 3 h after exposure to the stressor. In contrast, Maier et al. found that corticosterone values in rats exposed to escapable or inescapable shock declined in the same manner over time and approached baseline levels 2.5 h after shock exposure. These inconsistencies in the literature could reflect differences in the paradigms employed by the two research groups.

Tsuda and Tanaka (46) reported that 3 h and 6 h of yoked and escapable shock did not differentially affect corticosterone levels. Nevertheless, after repeated treatments over 5 consecutive days, animals in the yoked group exhibited significantly higher corticosterone concentrations than animals in the escape group. Although controllable and uncontrollable stressful situations appear to exert similar initial effects on the release of glucocorticoids, repeated uncontrollable stress treatments eventually produce higher corticosterone levels.

In dogs and rhesus monkeys (9,12), repeated treatment with uncontrollable stressors elevates cortisol levels relative to levels found in animals with control over the stressor. These findings are consistent with the research conducted in rats exposed repeatedly to uncontrollable stress and indicate that, under these circumstances, release of glucocorticoids provides sensitive physiological measures that reflect the degree of controllability.

Other studies have shown that corticosterone plays an important role in mediating analgesic effects produced by inescapable shock. Adrenalectomy blocks stress-induced analgesia induced by uncontrollable shock, and corticosterone replacement reinstates the analgesic response (29). Eliminating the release of corticosterone via ACTH secretion by hypophysectomy and dexamethasone treatment fails to reduce the behavioral depression shown in rats that have been subjected to inescapable shock (28). Collectively, these results show that some behavioral deficits produced by inescapable shock are not associated with decreases in pain sensitivity.

ATTACHMENT BOND DISRUPTION AND PROTEST-DESPAIR

Attachment bond disruption is a stressful event that occurs in the lives of human and nonhuman primates and other social species. Early work demonstrated that when human children are separated from their parents and placed in a nonsupportive environment, they respond acutely with behavioral agitation, disorganization, and decreased interest in their environment. As the separation continues, the agitation is replaced by behavioral inhibition and social withdrawal (3,42). A similar behavioral response occurs in some adults undergoing bereavement. Initially, behavioral disorganization and agitation occur. In some individuals this may progress to a depressive syndrome (27). Nonhuman primates in the wild exhibit similar responses to the disruption of attachment bonds (10,35), but in this situation the consequences of prolonged separation can be more profound, even resulting in death. Laboratory studies exploring this naturally occurring stressor have demonstrated that the disruption of attachment bonds in the mother-infant dyad of various primate species, including rhesus monkey peer groups, results in immediate behavioral alterations and activation of physiological and neuroendocrine systems (6,16,34,38). If the separation continues longer than 24 h, behavioral inhibition and withdrawal frequently occur (Fig. 2).

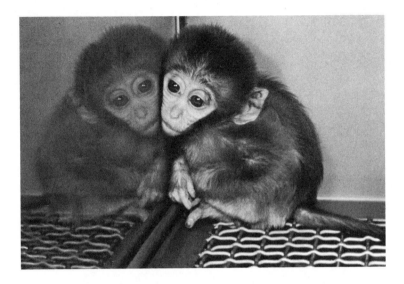

FIG. 2. Behavioral despair in an infant rhesus monkey separated from its mother.

Thus, various investigators have suggested that prolonged disruption of attachment bonds in nonhuman primates can serve as a model of depression (13,31). The tricyclic antidepressant imipramine significantly alleviates behavioral despair in separated rhesus monkeys (43), whereas agents that deplete brain catecholamines intensify separation-induced despair (23).

The effects of attachment bond disruption on HPA function have been investigated primarily in squirrel and rhesus monkeys. It is important to realize, however, that regulation of the HPA system in New World primates such as the squirrel monkey differs from that in Old World primates (rhesus monkey) and humans. New World primates have cortisol concentrations that are ten times higher and much less sensitive to the inhibitory effects of exogenously administered glucocorticoids (37). Consequently, similarities in regulation of the HPA axis in rhesus monkeys and humans make the rhesus monkey model particularly applicable to the understanding of depression in humans.

Brain CRH Systems

Corticotrophin-releasing hormone (CRH) and its receptors are distributed in hypothalamic and extrahypothalamic brain regions (8,47). Various lines of investigation have suggested that CRH neurons modulate and integrate the endocrine, autonomic, and behavioral consequences of exposure to stressors (4,5,24,36,44). Increased cerebrospinal fluid (CSF) concentrations of CRH occur in depressed patients (32), and research in animals suggests that when administered in high doses, CRH can result in behavioral inhibition (20) and abnormal self-directed behaviors (40).

To assess whether separation causes release of CRH into CSF, we measured CSF-CRH levels in infant monkeys after brief maternal separation. Concentrations of CRH were unaffected by separation. This result is consistent with our finding that CSF-CRH concentrations are not directly linked to pituitary-adrenal activity (unpublished data). Nevertheless, in earlier work, high doses of CRH administered intraventricularly to adult rhesus monkeys produced behavioral patterns characteristic of the despair response (Fig. 3). The same doses resulted in

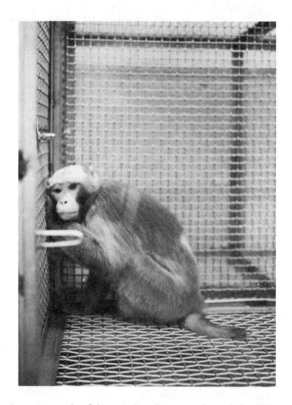

FIG. 3. Despair-like behavior produced by 20 μg of CRH administred intraventricularly to a rhesus monkey.

activation of ACTH and cortisol secretion. More recently, we administered lower doses of CRH intracerebrally (10 μg) to rhesus infants before separating them from their mothers. One hour after separation the monkeys were significantly less active than control monkeys given only the vehicle (unpublished data). A possible interpretation of these data is that the exogenously administered CRH caused a more rapid onset of behavioral patterns associated with behavioral depression or despair. Although further work is needed to confirm and extend these observations, our findings to date support a role of endogenous CRH systems in the pathophysiology of depression.

Brain and Pituitary ACTH

We are aware of no studies other than our own that have directly assessed the activation of ACTH secretion in relation to maternal separation. We recently performed studies in infant rhesus monkeys separated from their mothers for 1 hour (19 and unpublished data). Maternal separation induced the release of pituitary ACTH and adrenal cortisol but not prolactin (Fig. 4). We further demonstrated that opiates and benzodiazepines block this separation-induced release of ACTH (19), suggesting an involvement of endogenous opiate and benzodiazepine systems in this response.

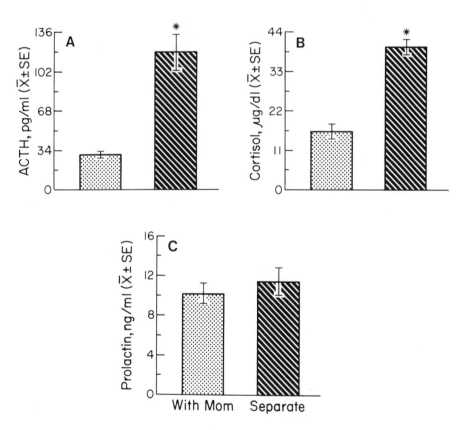

FIG. 4. Plasma concentrations of (A) ACTH, (B) cortisol, and (C) prolactin in 8 infant rhesus monkeys with their mothers (stippled bars) and 1 h after separation from their mothers (striped bars). * p ≤ .005.

The effects of prolonged separation in rhesus monkeys have also been examined. In these experiments, peer-housed juvenile monkeys that had formed stable attachment bonds to each other were separated. After four days of separation, plasma ACTH levels did not differ from preseparation levels, but CSF-ACTH concentrations increased significantly (15). This is of interest because CSF-ACTH likely reflects activity of brain ACTH neurons that are independent from pituitary ACTH and probably plays a role in regulating memory and behavior. Overall, our studies demonstrate that the acute response to separation results in an increased release of ACTH from the pituitary. After prolonged separation, plasma ACTH levels normalize but CSF levels increase.

Adrenal Cortisol Secretion

Cortisol has been the most extensively studied hormone in relation to separation. Studies in New World squirrel monkeys have shown repeatedly that plasma cortisol concentrations increase significantly in infants and mothers after separation (6,26,48). After repeated separation the cortisol response continues, whereas the behavioral response habituates.

In Old World monkeys, Smotherman et al. (41) found that cortisol concentrations significantly increased in rhesus infants 3 h after maternal separation. Gunnar et al. (11) studied nine rhesus mother-infant pairs separated for 12 days. They reported that cortisol concentrations in infant monkeys were significantly increased 30 min and 3 h after separation. However, 24 h after separation the cortisol levels had returned to normal and remained at baseline levels throughout the remainder of the extended separation. In this experiment the cortisol levels paralleled the degree of behavioral activation displayed by infants monkeys.

In other experiments we administered dexamethasone to rhesus monkeys 4 days after peer separation to assess HPA negative feedback insensitivity (22). In the first experiment, 4 of 11 monkeys changed from cortisol suppressors while living together to cortisol nonsuppressors during the separation period. In another study, eight monkeys were separated from each other and placed in a novel environment (21). The combination of novelty and separation elicited a qualitatively different behavioral response characterized by behavioral agitation and a high incidence of stereotypic behavior. In these animals we found a relationship between the observed amount of behavioral disturbance and the degree of cortisol nonsuppression. As shown in Fig. 5, animals that were extremely resistant to dexamethasone suppression (<20% decrease in cortisol concentrations after dexamethasone) displayed much more disturbance behavior than did the moderate nonsuppressors (<70% reduction of cortisol concentrations after dexamethasone). Animals that completely suppressed cortisol concentrations exhibited much less of the disturbance behavior.

In monkeys as in humans, an abnormal response to dexamethasone is not specific to separation-induced despair. We found that nonsuppression of cortisol can be produced in conditions other than attachment bond disruption. For example, individually housed monkeys placed in smaller novel cages exhibit resistance to dexamethasone (18).

The sensitivity of the HPA negative feedback system has also been studied in animals that had a history of exposure to stress but were not stressed at the time of dexamethasone administration (17). Here we modified the dexamethasone test using low doses that resulted in intermediate levels of cortisol suppression in nonstressed animals.

Consequently, an interesting relationship between the sensitivity of an individual animal's HPA feedback system and its prior degree of behavioral arousal to a stress was documented. Animals most responsive behaviorally to stressors early in life were also highly resistant to cortisol suppression after dexamethasone administration. These results suggest that the degree of HPA negative feedback sensitivity is an index of an animal's predisposition to stress-induced behavior.

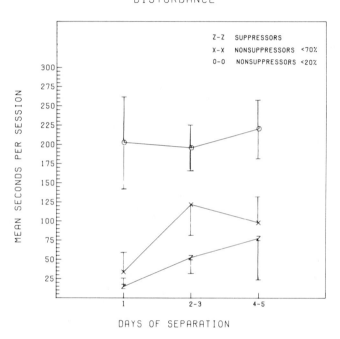

FIG. 5. Disturbance behaviors seen in rhesus monkeys after peer separation in relation to dexamethasone suppression of cortisol.

Few studies have examined the direct effect of HPA manipulations on the separation response. Dexamethasone administration has been reported to result in a rapid cessation of distress vocalizations without affecting activity levels in infant squirrel monkeys separated from their mothers. The mechanism underlying these effects is not clear, because dexamethasone suppresses both plasma ACTH and cortisol. Metyrapone inhibits adrenal cortical enzymes essential for the synthesis of cortisol, resulting in extremely low cortisol concentrations with subsequent increases in plasma ACTH concentrations. Metyrapone administered to separated infant squirrel monkeys has been reported to decrease activity and, in a few individuals, to elicit body postures characteristic of behavioral depression (7).

SUMMARY AND CONCLUSIONS

Exposure to uncontrollable stress and the disruption of attachment bonds can alter the regulation of the HPA system. Although one exposure to an uncontrollable shock schedule does not result in differential release of ACTH between animals receiving escapable or yoked inescapable shock, repeated exposure to uncontrollable shock enhances the secretion of ACTH. In the separation paradigm, an immediate release of pituitary ACTH occurs after separation, but ACTH normalizes after several days. However, after prolonged separation, CSF-ACTH concentrations are higher than preseparation levels. This finding implicates activation of brain ACTH neurons in the despair response.

Glucocorticoid levels increase acutely in both paradigms. After repeated sessions of uncontrollable shock glucocorticoid levels are higher than in animals treated with repeated controllable shock. Similarly, glucocorticoid values increase after separation in both Old and New World monkeys. As the separation continues the glucocorticoid levels normalize. In studies with rhesus monkeys, HPA negative feedback insensitivity develops in some animals after prolonged separation.

Few studies have directly assessed the role of HPA hormones in mediating learned helplessness and the effects of attachment bond disruption. Activation of brain CRH systems in monkeys results in behavioral patterns that are also observed during separation-induced despair. In addition, monkeys undergoing brief separation develop behavioral inhibition after CRH infusion into the brain. The CRH system remains to be studied in relation to learned helplessness.

The specific role of ACTH is not clear because direct experimental manipulations often affect both adrenal glucocorticoids and pituitary ACTH. In monkeys, preliminary studies suggest that dexamethasone decreases separation-induced vocalizations. Metyrapone administration, which results in decreased cortisol and increased ACTH, appears to exacerbate behavioral inhibition during separation. Evidence suggests that corticosterone modulates the development of analgesia, but not behavioral depression, in rats exposed to inescapable shock.

LITERATURE CITED

1. Anisman, H., Pizzino, A., and Sklar, L.S. (1980): Brain Res., 191: 583-588.
2. Anisman, H., Suissa, A., and Sklar, L.S. (1980): Behav. Neur. Biol., 28:34-37.
3. Bowlby, J. (1980): Psychoanal. Study Child, 15:9-52.
4. Britton, K.T., Lee, G., Vale, W., Rivier, J., and Koob, G.F. (1986): Brain Res., 369:303-306.
5. Brown, M.R., Fisher, L.A., Rivier, J., Spiess, J., Rivier, C., and Vale, W. (1982): Life Sci., 30:207-210.
6. Coe, C.L., Mendoza, S.P., Smotherman, W.P., and Levine, S. (1978): Behav. Biol., 22:256-263.
7. Coe, C.L., Wiener, S.G., Rosenberg, L.T. (1985): In: The Psychobiology of Attachment and Separation, edited by M. Reite and T. Field, pp. 163-199, Academic Press, New York.
8. De Souza, E.B., Perrin, M.H., Insel, T.R., Rivier, J., Vale, W.W., and Kuhar, M.J. (1984): Science, 224:1449-1451.
9. Dess, N.K., Linwick, D., Patterson, J., Overmeier, J.B., and Levine, S. (1983): Behav. Neurosci., 97:1005-1016.

10. Goodall, J. (1979): Natl. Geogr., 155:592-620.
11. Gunnar, M.R., Gonzalez, C.A., Goodlin, B.L., and Levine, S. (1981): Psychoneuroendocrinology, 6:65-75.
12. Hanson, J.D., Larson, M.E., and Snowdon, C.T. (1976): Behav. Biol., 16:333-340.
13. Harlow, H.F., and Suomi, S.J. (1974): Behav. Biol., 12:273-296.
14. Jackson, R.L., Maier, S.F., and Coon, D.J. (1979): Science, 206: 91-93.
15. Kalin, N.H. (1986): Biol. Psychiatry, 21:124-140.
16. Kalin, N.H., and Carnes, M. (1984): Neuropsychopharmacol. Biol. Psychiatry, 8:459-469.
17. Kalin, N.H., Cohen, R.M., Kraemer, G.W., Risch, S.C., Shelton, S.E., Cohen, M., McKinney, W.T., and Murphy, D.L. (1981): Neuro-endocrinology, 32:92-95.
18. Kalin, N.H., and Shelton, S.E. (1984): Biol. Psychiatry, 19: 113-117.
19. Kalin, N.H., Shelton, S.E., and Barksdale, C.M. (1987): Brain Res. (in press).
20. Kalin, N.H., Shelton, S.E., Kraemer, G.W., and McKinney, W.T. (1983): Peptides, 4:217-220.
21. Kalin, N.H., Shelton, S.E., McKinney, W.T., Kraemer, G.W., Scanlon, J., and Suomi, S.J. (1983): Psychopharmacol. Bull., 19:542-544.
22. Kalin, N.H., Weiler, S.J., McKinney, W.T., Kraemer, G.W., and Shelton, S.E. (1982): Psychopharmacol. Bull., 18:219-222.
23. Kraemer, G.W., and McKinney, W.T. (1979): J. Affect. Disord., 1: 33-54.
24. Krahn, D.D., Gosnell, B.A., Grace, M., and Levine, A.S. (1986): Brain Res. Bull., 17:285-289.
25. Laudenslager, M.L., Ryan, S.M., Drugan, R.C., Hyson, R.L., and Maier, S.F. (1983): Science, 221:568-570.
26. Levine, S., Coe, C.L., Smotherman, W.P., and Kaplan, J.N. (1978): Physiol. Behav., 20:7-10.
27. Lindemann, E. (1944): Psychiatry, 101:141-148.
28. MacLennan, A.J., Drugan, R.C., Hyson, R.L., Maier, S.F., Madden, J., IV, and Barchas, J.D. (1982): J. Comp. Physiol. Psychol., 96: 904-912.
29. MacLennan, A.J., Drugan, R.L., Hyson, R.L., Maier, S.F., Madden, J., IV, and Barchas, J.D. (1982): Science, 215:1530-1532.
30. Maier, S.F., Ryan, S.M., Barksdale, C.M., and Kalin, N.H. (1986): Behav. Neurosci., 100:669-674.
31. McKinney, W.T. (1972): In: Animal Models in Psychiatry and Neurology, edited by I. Hanin and E. Usdin, pp. 117-126, Pergamon Press, New York.
32. Nemeroff, C.B., Widerlov, E., Bissette, G., Walleus, H., Karlsson, I., Eklund, K., Kilts, C.D., Loosen, P.T., and Vale, W. (1984): Science, 226:1342-1344.
33. Overmeier, J.B., and Seligman, M.E.P. (1967): J. Comp. Physiol. Psychol., 63:23-33.
34. Reite, M., and Short, R.A. (1978): Arch. Gen. Psychiatry, 35: 1247-1253.
35. Rhine, R.J., Norton, G.W., Roertgen, W.J., and Klein, H.D. (1980): Int. J. Primatol., 1:401-409.
36. Rivier, C., and Vale, W. (1983): Nature, 305:325-327.
37. Sapolsky, R.M., Krey, L.C., and McEwen, B.S. (1986): Endocrine Rev., 7:284-301.

38. Seay, B., Hansen, E., and Harlow, H. (1962): J. Child Psychol. Psychiatry, 3:123-132.
39. Seligman, M.E.P., and Maier, S.F. (1967): J. Exp. Psychol., 74: 1-9.
40. Sherman, J.E., and Kalin, N.H. (1986): Life Sci., 39:433-441.
41. Smotherman, W.P., Hunt, L.E., McGinnis, L.M., and Levine, S. (1979): Dev. Psychobiol., 12:211-217.
42. Spitz, R.A. (1946): Psychoanal. Study Child, 2:313-342.
43. Suomi, S.J., Seaman, S.F., Lewis, J.K., Delizio, R.D., and McKinney, W.T. (1978): Arch. Gen. Psychiatry, 35:321-325.
44. Sutton, R.E., Koob, G.F., LeMoal, M., Rivier, J., and Vale, W. (1982): Nature, 297:331-335.
45. Swenson, R.M., and Vogel, W.H. (1983): Pharmacol. Biochem. Behav., 18:689-693.
46. Tsuda, A., and Tanaka, M. (1985): Behav. Neurosci., 99:802-817.
47. Vale, W., Rivier, C., Brown, M., Plotsky, P., Smith, M., Bilezikjian, L., Bruhn, T., Perrin, M., Spiess, J., and Rivier, J. (1984): In: Secretory Tumors of the Pituitary Gland, Progress in Endocrine Research and Therapy, edited by P. McL. Black et al., pp. 213-225, Raven Press, New York.
48. Vogt, J.L., Levine, S. (1980): Physiol. Behav., 24:829-832.
49. Weinberg, J., and Levine, S. (1980): In: Coping and Health, edited by S. Levine and H. Ursin, pp. 39-59, Plenum Press, New York.
50. Weiss, J.M. (1971): J. Comp. Physiol. Psychol., 77:1-13.
51. Weiss, J.M. (1971): J. Comp. Physiol. Psychol., 77:22-30.
52. Weiss, J.M., Bailey, W.H., Pohorecky, L.A., Korzeniowski, D., and Grillone, G. (1980): Neurochem. Res., 5:9-22.

The Hypothalamic-Pituitary-Adrenal Axis:
Physiology, Pathophysiology, and Psychiatric
Implications, edited by A.F. Schatzberg and
C.B. Nemeroff. Raven Press, Ltd., New York
© 1988.

HUMAN CORTICOTROPIN-RELEASING HORMONE CHALLENGE TESTS IN DEPRESSION

F.Holsboer, U.von Bardeleben, I. Heuser, A. Steiger

Department of Psychiatry, University of Mainz,
6500 Mainz, FRG

INTRODUCTION

The recent sequencing and subsequent synthesis of ovine-cortico-tropin-releasing hormone (o-CRH) by Vale et al. (1) and its human analogue (h-CRH) by Shibahara et al. (2) opened the possibility to study pathophysiology underlying various aberrancies of the pituitary-adrenocortical system in the affective disorders. Since hypersecretion of corticosteroids represents one of the most extensively studied abnormalities in affective disorders it was intended to investigate by means of o- and h-CRH infusions, if hypercortisolemia linked to depression can be attributed to a limbic-hypothalamic disturbance. Clarification of this point would be of importance since biological markers of psychiatric illness which were derived from limbic-hypothalamic-pituitary-adrenocortical (LHPA)-function should rather be related to a central nervous system disturbance than to a peripheral abnormality. Because o-CRH was discovered and synthesized first the initial studies in affectively ill patients from our group and other investigators used this heterologous peptide whose pharmacological properties are substantially different from those of the human analogue (3,4). Both peptides proved to be equally potent in their ability to stimulate maximal ACTH secretion but the homologous (human) hormone (h-CRH) has a reported half-time of serum disappearance (first phase) of about 9 minutes, which is significantly less than that of an ovine analogue (18 minutes). This difference results in broader ACTH peaks than spontaneous physiologic bursts while so far no appreciable advantage of o-CRH compared with h-CRH was reported. Theoretically, h-CRH bears several advantages for clinical application because it has no antigenic property. Therefore, we conducted a series of studies using the homologous h-CRH as soon as it became available for clinical research. These investigations intended to unravel pathophysiology of altered LHPA function in patients with affective disorders and related illness rather than establishing a diagnostic test.

ACTH AND CORTISOL RESPONSE TO h-CRH IN MAJOR ENDOGENOUS DEPRESSION AND NORMAL CONTROLS (5,6)

Eleven depressed patients (4 m, 7 f, age: 42-62 yrs, mean $\pm$ SD: 52.1 $\pm$ 7.0) who met research diagnostic criteria (RDC)(7) for major depressive disorder and DSM-III criteria for major depressive episode (n=9) or bipolar disorder, depressed (n=2), were enrolled to the study. All investigations were performed after the nature of the protocol was fully explained and voluntary informed consent was obtained. All subjects underwent a rigid medical investigation including studies of

endocrine status to exclude factors that could invalidate the study
results. Prior to investigation a drug free period of at least 14 days
was initiated. Hamilton Rating Scale (HRS) scores ranged between 18-30
points (mean $\pm$ SD: 24.1 $\pm$ 4.4). Eleven normal control subjects (7 m, 4
f, age: 23-62 yrs, mean $\pm$ SD: 38.9 $\pm$ 11.2) participated on a paid
voluntary basis after written informed consent was obtained and after
all contaminants (alcohol or coffeine abuse, time shifts, sleep deprivation, stressfull life-events, medical illness, drug intake etc) which
could render an endocrine evaluation ambiguous were carefully ruled
out. Their body weights were 69.6$\pm$ 9.0 kg and thus not statistically
different from those of the depressed patients (73.6 $\pm$ 8.9 kg). All
subjects received a standard diet designed to keep electrolytes and
calories constant at 7:00 am and 11:30 am. At 1:00 pm, an indwelling
venous catheter was inserted into a forearm vein and kept patent with
slow normal saline infusion (50 ml/h). The subjects were resting supine
in bed in a separate room while observed on a television screen located
in the adjacent laboratory. The catheter was connected to a long tube
and passed from the patient's room into the neighboring laboratory.
There, blood samples for cortisol determinations were obtained every 30
minutes until 7:00 pm and additional baseline samples for ACTH were
collected at 6:30 pm, 6:45 pm and 7:00 pm. At 7:00 pm 100 ug of h-CRH
dissolved in 1 ml 0.02% HCl in 0.9% saline was infused directly into
the cannula within 30 sec. Following h-CRH infusion, samples for ACTH
and cortisol determinations were drawn every 15 minutes until 8:00 pm
and every 30 min until 11:00 pm.
The h-CRH lot (Bissendorf-Peptide, Wedemark, FRG) was analysed by high
pressure liquid chromatography to determine the purity of the peptide
preparation which has proven to be above 98.5%. This synthetic peptide
was lyophilized in sterile ampoules by aliquotation which resulted in a
precision of 100 $\pm$ 3% for the 100 ug vials employed in the current
studies. Each blood sample was collected into chilled tubes, which contained heparine for cortisol or ethylenediaminetetraacetate (1mg/ml)
and 400 KIU trasylol/ml for ACTH determinations. Plasma was promptly
separated by centrifugation at 4°C and stored at -80°C. Cortisol determinations were performed by radioimmunoassay (Gammacoat, Travenol). The
precision criteria (intraassay variation =4-7% and interassay variation
5-8%) of this method are routinely monitored longitudinally to exclude
batch to batch variation. The ACTH-antiserum used in this study is
specifically N-terminal and requires preceding plasma extraction using
silica-gel. The extraction yield, when applying a 125-I-ACTH (1-39)
tracer was 75% with a coefficient of variation (CV) less than 2%. The
intraassay CV in the middle range of the standard curve was 6.4%. At
the lower limit of detection (5-10 pg/ml) the CV increased to values
below 20%. The assay does not significantly cross-react with α , ß-, y-
endorphins or ß-lipotropin.
This experimental setting was maintained in all the studies reported
here and is referred to as standard h-CRH test.

As illustrated in Fig.1 h-CRH administration prompted a marked increase of ACTH and cortisol. ACTH secretion following a bolus of 100 ug
h-CRH at 7:00 pm was significantly blunted in depressives when compared with controls. This difference is also documented by calculated
areas under time course curves (AUC) where the net ACTH output for
depressives was 3.0 $\pm$ 2.6 pg x min/ml$\cdot$ 10^3 and for controls 6.2 $\pm$ 3.4
pg x min/ml$\cdot$ 10^3 (t=2.4, df=20, p$<$0.05; U=21, p$<$0.01). Mean cortisol

secretion between 2 pm and 7 pm was significantly higher in depressives than in controls (95.3 ± 25.8 ng/ml versus 56.6 ± 14.6 ng/ml, t=4.3, df=20, p < 0.001). However, net cortisol release following h-CRH resulted in indistinguishable cortisol responses (11.5 ± 4.2 ng x min/ml·10^3 versus 11.8 ± 4.6 ng x min/ml· 10^3, p = ns). The high baseline cortisol secretory activity was found to be associated with blunted ACTH output after h-CRH because a significant negative correlation between these two measures has been found (r=-0.48, p < 0.05). Our observation of blunted ACTH and normal cortisol response to h-CRH in patients with

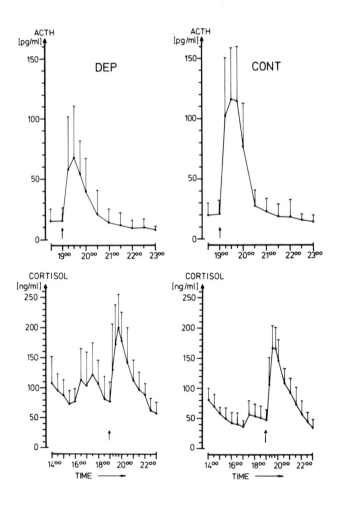

Fig. 1

ACTH and cortisol (Mean ± SD) release before and following a bolus of 100 ug h-CRH (7 pm, arrow) to patients with endogenous depression (n=11) and to normal controls (n=11). From Holsboer et al. (6)

depression is compatible with the following mechanism:
Hypersecretion of CRH from the nucleus paraventricularis into hypophyseal portal vessels increases ACTH and cortisol concentrations. Elevated glucocorticoid levels and endogenous CRH overstimulation resulting in down-regulation of CRH receptors at corticotrophic pituitary cells reduce their capacity to release ACTH after specific stimulation with exogenous h-CRH. This feedback regulation restrains adequate ACTH response in depressives with elevated circulating cortisol levels.Persistent LHPA overactivity leads primarily to elevated levels of circulating ACTH, which is a trophic hormone inducing a mild functional hyperplasia of the adrenocortex. Such a phenomenon is also present in endocrine diseases associated with ACTH excess, e.g. congenital adrenal hyperplasia and would explain why in depressives less ACTH after h-CRH is sufficient to produce cortisol output being indistinguishable from normals.
These studies provide the first experimental evidence to support the hypothesis that LHPA-hyperactivity in depression originates from pathology in the CNS and are in agreement with parallel studies by Gold et al. who employed the long acting ovine analogue of h-CRH (8,9).

DIFFERENTIAL MINERALOCORTICOID AND GLUCOCORTICOID RELEASE FOLLOWING h-CRH IN DEPRESSION (10)

Several previous investigations indicated that mineralocorticoid homeostasis is disturbed in depression. Hullin et al. (11) reported that in vitro production of aldosterone is altered if adrenocortical cell cultures were exposed to sera of patients during depression when contrasted to effects by sera collected during the manic state. Our group has first demonstrated that aldosterone increases following dexamethasone are blunted in depression (12). Despite increasing evidence that aldosterone is regulated partly by ACTH-independent processes, h-CRH proved to be a stimulus for the mineralocorticoids deoxycorticosterone and aldosterone (13). Here we report a comparative evaluation of ACTH cortisol and aldosterone responses to h-CRH in depressives and matched controls. We also used corticosterone as an additional reference hormone because we detected recently that this steroid, which is pharmacologically a glucocorticoid but is synthesized via the mineralocorticoid pathway, responds most sensitively among all so far tested corticosteroids to an ovine or h-CRH challenge.

Ten psychiatric inpatients (5 m, 5 f; age: 40 - 62 ; mean $\pm$ SD: 48.8 $\pm$ 7) suffering from a major depressive episode according to the DSM-III classification and 10 individually matched controls were admitted. All subjects were carefully examined for medical factors that could invalidate study results. These investigations included an endocrine evaluation, determination of electrolytes in plasma and 24-hour urine collections, confirmation of present normotension and absence of past history or family history of hypertension, abuse of coffeine containing beverages and intake of any kind of drugs. A h-CRH bolus of 100 ug was administered in the standard route as described above.

The net hormone responses are illustrated in Fig. 2. They show that aldosterone responses to h-CRH were significantly blunted in depressives, whereas cortisol and corticosterone output was unaltered.

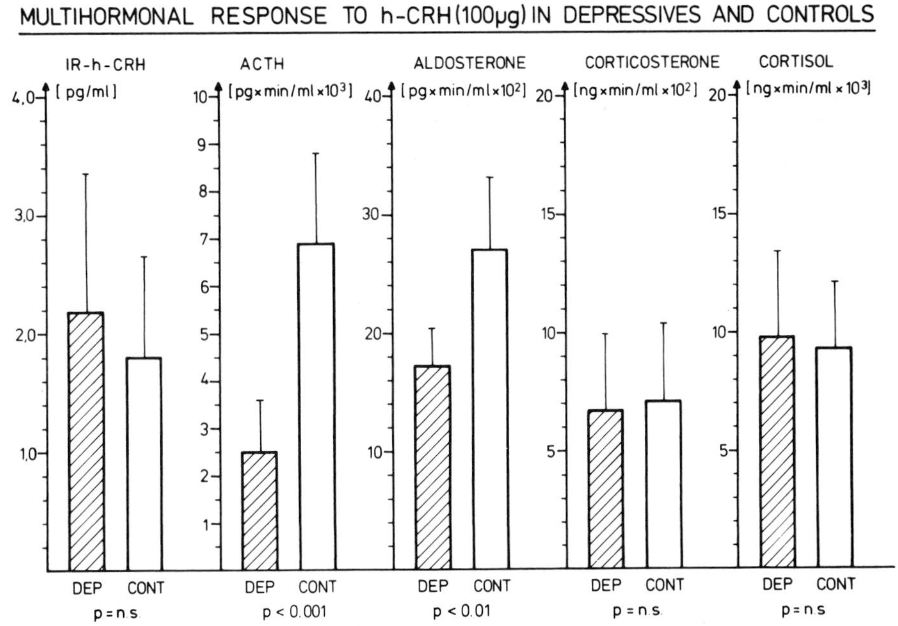

MULTIHORMONAL RESPONSE TO h-CRH (100μg) IN DEPRESSIVES AND CONTROLS

Fig. 2

Multihormonal response to h-CRH in 10 patients (PAT) with MDE and 10 matched controls (CON) revealed significantly lowered ACTH and aldosterone responses in depressives, but normal responses of both glucocorticoids, cortisol and corticosterone. From Holsboer et al. (10).

This observation adds to earlier reports of disturbed electrolyte homeostasis in patients with affective disorders which was related to impaired aldosterone production rates (11). One clue for understanding differential glucocorticoid and mineralocorticoid responses in relation to ACTH following h-CRH is the detection that adrenal steroid receptor systems in the brain are diversified (14). If corroborated in larger study samples under various clinical conditions including drug status the finding of altered mineralocorticosteroid function may provide a basis to understand vulnerability of patients with affective disorders to suffer from kidney pathology, particularly if treated with lithium.

EFFECT OF DEXAMETHASONE PRETREATMENT ON ACTH AND CORTISOL
RESPONSE TO h-CRH IN DEPRESSIVES AND CONTROLS (15,16)

Nonsuppression of ACTH and cortisol after a dexamethasone suppression test (DST) was originally regarded as a peripheral outprint of a centrally mediated overdrive of CRH. In order to test this hypothesis we further explored the pathophysiology underlying DST-nonsuppression. We compared pituitary-adrenal response to placebo, h-CRH or lysine-vasopressin (LVP) with a concurrent application of both neuropeptides in 6 normal controls pretreated with 1.5 mg dexamethasone.

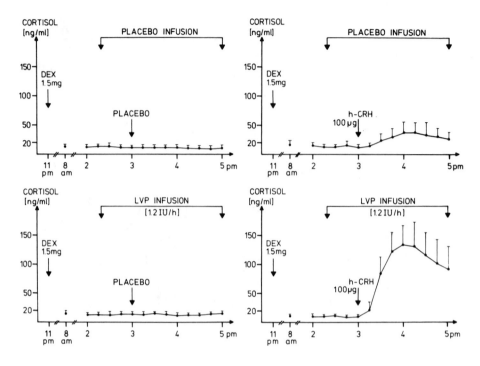

Fig. 3

Plasma cortisol concentrations (mean ± SD) collected from 6 male controls after 1.5 mg dexamethasone at 11 pm, and following infusions of placebo, h-CRH, LVP and combinations hereof at time points as indicated. From von Bardeleben et al. (15).

Infusion of LVP (1.2 IU/h) given in the afternoon failed to provoke ACTH and cortisol elevation (Fig. 3). Also a h-CRH bolus (100 ug) administered at 3:00 pm induced only a modest release of ACTH and cortisol above hormone levels observed after placebo infusion. However, if both peptides were administered in combination a substantial escape of plasma cortisol from dexamethasone suppression became apparent. Since ACTH levels increased in parallel with cortisol it was concluded that LVP synergizes the effect of h-CRH at pituitary-corticotrophs to override dexamethasone suppression. This allows us to hypothesize that CRH overproduction is not the only mechanism to explain DST resistance and suggests that other factors including synergizing neuropeptides, altered activity of neural efferent pathways and changes at feedback receptor levels are corequired. In line with this contention is a recent study by Nemeroff et al. (17) who measured CRH in cerebrospinal fluid and observed elevated levels in major depression which were not related to the DST status.
Based on these findings obtained from normal controls we embarked on a series of clinical studies applying a combined DST/CRH-test to patients with major depressive episodes which were repeatedly studied during the course of their illness and following clinical recovery (16). Four patients with a DSM-III diagnosis of major depressive episode either bipolar (n=1) or unipolar (n=3) were studied first after a drug-free

period of 8-12 days and hereafter three to four times during a course of tricyclic antidepressant treatment. They received a DST (oral dose of 1.5 mg at 11 pm) and were challenged with a bolus of 100 ug h-CRH at 3:00 pm applying the standard experimental design.

We classified three patients as DST nonsuppressors at the first test. After h-CRH administration all subjects responded with a release of ACTH and cortisol. At the second test two patients had changes in their DST status (one from suppression to nonsuppression, and one from nonsuppression to suppression) while all four responded with an increase of ACTH and cortisol after h-CRH (two of these cases are illustrated in Fig. 4). All patients became DST suppressors at the third test and h-CRH-induced escape from suppression was observable in only one case. Three patients were retested for a fourth time, while they were DST suppressors. Two of them showed a moderate elevation of ACTH and cortisol after ACTH. This gradual reduction of releasable ACTH and cortisol after h-CRH was associated with clinical improvement or a switch into mania (Fig. 4, bottom). One patient who showed a failure of dexamethasone to inhibit h-CRH induced cortisol elevation at the fourth test needed rehospitalization because of a relapse occurring several weeks after discharge. Since we recently demonstrated an association between DST nonsuppression of cortisol and low plasma dexamethasone levels (18) we ruled out that individual ACTH and cortisol responses were an artifact of inadequate dexamethasone absorption as we measured comparable amounts of the test drug in the plasma samples at 8 am in all patients at all test occasions. All patients maintained their initial tricyclic treatment and had comparable plasma levels throughout the study, thus excluding different drug plasma concentrations confounding study results.

The principal finding of the present study is that in depressed patients ACTH and cortisol were releasable after h-CRH administration despite dexamethasone pretreatment. This phenomenon disappeared if depressive symptomatology resolved or switched into mania and persisted in one patient being at risk for a clinical relapse into depression. Interestingly, the ability of h-CRH to enhance ACTH and cortisol release was independent from DST status.

While dexamethasone was sufficiently potent to inhibit pituitary-adrenal stimulation by h-CRH in normal controls (15) this was not the case in the investigated four patients during a depressive episode. This comes as a surprise since in altogether six tests the elevation of ACTH and cortisol after h-CRH was associated with DST nonsuppression prior to stimulation. In these cases both dexamethasone and exogenous elevated endogenous corticosteroids failed to inhibit stimulatory effects of h-CRH at the pituitary level.

One possible mechanism involved in the current observation implies glucocorticoid receptor changes. Tornello et al. (19) demonstrated that exogenous administration of glucocorticoids reduces cytosolic glucocorticoid receptor number in the hippocampus which is an important element for the negative feedback loop of the limbic-hypothalamic-pituitary-adrenocortical (LHPA) system (20).Another recent study (21) showed that repeated stress given to rats reduces the number of glucocorticoid receptors in various brain structures including the hippocampus (21). If glucocorticoid hypersecretion during depression continues a stepwise reduction in hippocampal corticosteroid receptor number could develop which results in reduced sensitivity of this feedback element toward circulating corticosteroids. Administration of dexamethasone

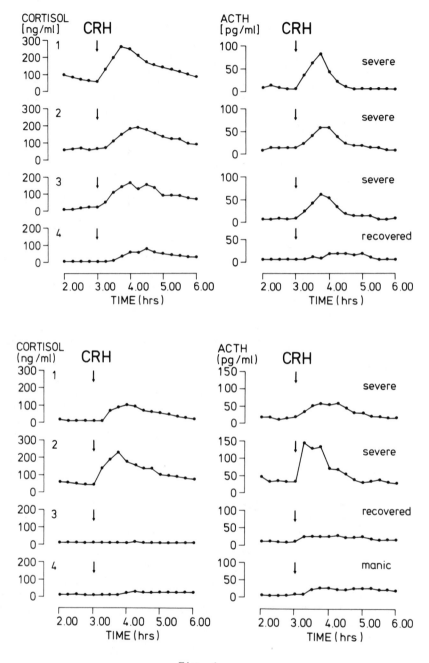

Fig. 4

Serial applications of combined DST/CRH-tests to
patients with endogenous depression show a gradual
return from abnormal cortisol and ACTH surges
during the depressive state to normal nonresponse
after clinical improvement or a switch into mania.
From Holsboer et al. (16).

results mainly in occupation of pituitary glucocorticoid receptors reducing ACTH and corticosteroid release. At the level of the hippocampus this withdrawal of endogenous corticosteroids is not compensated by dexamethasone since in comparison to pituitary corticotrophic binding its retention by limbic neurons particularly in the hippocampus is different from that of naturally occurring glucocorticoids (14). The pharmacologic effect of dexamethasone administration upon hippocampal sites can thus be described as a "chemical adrenalectomy" to which hippocampal neurons respond with enhanced activation of the LHPA system. Following dexamethasone, the amount of ACTH which is finally released at baseline or after stimulation with h-CRH depends upon the equilibrium of enforcing (via hippocampus) and suppressing (via pituitary) inputs upon the entire system. In depression, persistent elevation of corticosteroids may increase vulnerability of glucocorticosteroid receptor containing cells at hippocampal and other central sites. This effect weakens the negative feedback system making the corticotropic cells more susceptible to stimuli such as h-CRH. After dexamethasone administration the reduced glucocorticosteroid receptor population is no longer capable to inhibit LHPA activation which then can override the suppressive effect of dexamethasone at corticotropic cells.

In these cases endogenous corticosteroids in combination with exogenous dexamethasone are not sufficient to serve as a brake for additional pituitary-adrenal activation after h-CRH. When central regulation returns to normalcy there is a stepwise increase of receptor sensitivity resulting in an adrenocortical response to h-CRH which is indistinguishable from that in normal controls. In cases where sustained hypercortisolism has produced neuronal loss in central feedback elements, altered pituitary-adrenal activity would persist. This mechanism may also account for increased pituitary-adrenocortical activity associated with growing age.

Because of the small number of subjects included in this study the present observations and conclusions are preliminary and warrant corroboration in larger studies. Our current data base on the combined DST/CRH test holds promise to uncover important features of DST refractoriness and further supports a central pathophysiology underlying altered LHPA function in a subset of depressives.

EFFECT OF LONG TERM CARBAMAZEPINE TREATMENT UPON ACTH AND CORTISOL RELEASE AFTER h-CRH

Carbamazepine, which is expected to enter clinical routine as a prophylactic and possibly also as an acute treatment of bipolar disorder interferes with LHPA physiology. To further explore this phenomenon we conducted standard h-CRH tests in 6 asymptomatic depressives (4 f, 2 m; age: 26-54; duration of carbamazepine-treatment 2-27 months; maintenance dosage: 300-1600 ug/d; plasma drug level 5-8 mg/l) during long-term carbamazepine treatment. We observed highly exaggerated ACTH responses in 2 patients accompanied with high baseline and peak cortisol response in one of these cases, while in the other case exaggerated ACTH output was associated with normal cortisol release (Fig. 5). There is no ready answer for these aberrant corticotrophic cell responses, since demographic and clinical characteristics were not different among the study subjects. Also the failure of adequate cortisol response following excessive ACTH remains unclear and probably supports that immunoreactive ACTH which is measured by radioimmunoassay contains a fraction of biologically inactive ACTH in these two patients.

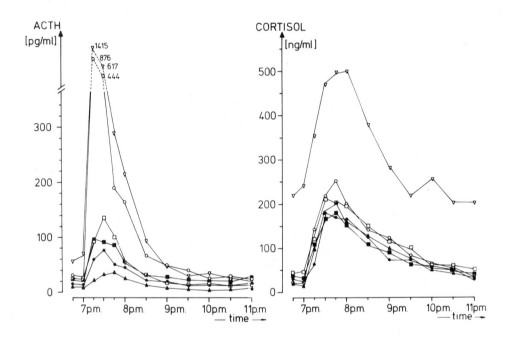

Fig. 5

ACTH and cortisol response in 6 asymptomatic patients with major depression during long-term treatment with carbamazepine. While 4 patients show normal (Mean $\pm$SEM is expressed as shaded area) ACTH responses to h-CRH, excessive immunoreactive ACTH output was measured in two other patients.

Serby et al.(22) recently proposed that somatostatin may be involved in the regulation of the LHPA-axis, because somatostatin was significantly negatively correlated with post-DST cortisol levels in demented men. This intriguing hypothesis is supported by our present data since carbamazepine may reduce CSF somatostatin in a subset of patients during long term treatment (23). The clinical relevance of this finding is that selected patients treated with carbamazepine develop altered LHPA function, which in turn may influence clinical course (24).

ACTH AND CORTISOL RESPONSE TO h-CRH IN ALCOHOL WITHDRAWAL

In patients with alcoholism several abnormalities of LHPA-function are well documented (25, 26). However, it remained unclear, whether hypercortisolism in these patients results from an abnormality at a limbic-hypothalamic or pituitary-adrenocortex site. To further elucidate alcohol-induced alteration of LHPA physiology we performed standard h-CRH tests in eight unmedicated patients (age:20-48 yrs) who were acutely withdrawn from excessive alcohol consumption. They were compared with eight sex matched healthy controls (age: 24-48 yrs). Figure 6 shows that ACTH responses were significantly lower (mean area under-time-course curves in patients: 1.6 ± 1.0 pg x min/ml $\cdot$ 10^3; in controls: 5.5 ± 3.0 pg x min/ml $\cdot 10^3$, $t = 3.0$, $df = 14$, $p < 0.01$). Cortisol output was less marked in patients with alcoholism (6.8 ± 4.3 ng x min/ml $\cdot 10^3$ versus 11.8 ± 4.2 ng x min/ml $\cdot$ 10^3, $t = 2.3$, $p < 0.05$). Mean cortisol secretion before stimulation was higher in the patients than in controls (105.4 ± 48 ng/ml vs 55.6 ± 24.7, $t = 3.0$, $p < 0.01$). The mechanism for this restrained ACTH release may be explained as follows: Ethanol centrally enhances the release of CRH which in turn leads to hypersecretion of ACTH and subsequently of cortisol. Increased glucocorticoid levels and CRH stimulation may also down regulate CRH receptors at corticotrophic cells attenuating CRH stimulated ACTH secretion. Additionally, chronic ethanol exposure to rats decreases CRH pituitary binding and reduces POMC mRNA levels (27). These mechanisms may act in concert to reduce pituitary corticotrophic cell response to exogenous h-CRH. In comparison to ACTH the cortisol responses are less

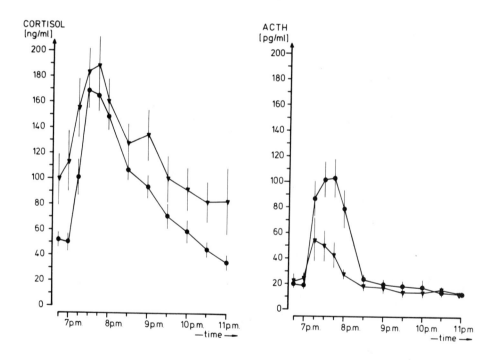

Fig. 6

ACTH and cortisol responses to 100 ug CRH in 8 patients during acute alcohol withdrawal (closed triangles) and 8 normal matched controls (closed circles).

blunted in alcohol abstinence which suggests the development of a functional hyperplasia of the adrenocortex resulting from sustained ACTH hypersecretion. However, other ACTH-independent mechanisms may also be effective.

Whether similar hormonal response patterns after h-CRH in patients with alcoholism and depression are a possible link to their reported genetic proximity remains a hypothesis worthy to be tested.

APPLICATION OF HETEROLOGOUS OVINE CRH TO DIFFERENTIATE PATIENTS WITH CUSHING'S DISEASE FROM NORMAL CONTROLS AND PATIENTS WITH DEPRESSION

As demonstrated by several authors (9,28) most patients with Cushing's disease respond to o-CRH with exaggerated ACTH output, despite high baseline cortisol levels. This response pattern allows the clinical differentiation between Cushing's syndrome due to ectopic ACTH production where high ACTH titers are nonresponsive to h-CRH and Cushing's disease due to an autonomous ACTH-dependent pituitary adenoma. Ovine CRH-tests can be helpful to differentiate between primary depression with hypercortisolism and mild Cushing's disease which is frequently associated with mood disorder (9).

We confirmed that patients with Cushing's disease in general have an ACTH response to o-CRH which is clearly distinct from that observed in normal controls and patients with endogenous depression (29). It should be noted however, that ACTH response to o-CRH is highly variable in Cushing's disease, where some patients remain even totally refractory to the specific stimulus. Also the diagnostic specificity of the o-CRH test to differentiate between Cushing's disease and depression remains to be evaluated because a recent investigation showed that 20 percent of depressives have ACTH peaks in the range of responses of the patients with Cushing's disease and 27 percent of patients with Cushing's disease responded similarly to depressives (9). While the diagnostic characterization of Cushing's syndromes benefited greatly from CRH-tests this endocrine intervention does not clarify the etiology of pituitary-dependent Cushing's disease. A hypothesis of central origin, as proposed by Krieger can not be ultimately rejected as primary pathogenetic cause of Cushing's disease. Some recent evidence from van Cauter and Refetoff (30) also supports the existence of a "hypothalamic hyperpulsative" type of Cushing's disease. These considerations are of psychiatric interest, because our group as well as other investigators proposed that Cushing's disease associated with affective symptomatology and major depression associated with hypercortisolism can be located at the opposite sites of a continuum characterized by LHPA-overactivity (31). As shown in Fig. 7 these two clinical states can be frequently distinguished from each other with the o-CRH test, because only depressives but not patients with Cushing's disease have an intact feedback circuitry between pituitary and adrenocortex. This test, when performed with o-CRH in the morning, however, did not allow us to distinguish between normals and depressives in a similar way as the studies conducted in the evening employing human-CRH (5,6,10). Also no differences in the net ACTH secretion between depressed DST suppressors and nonsuppressors (32) or patients during depression and after clinical recovery were observed (33) when the o-CRH challenge test was performed in morning. Apparently, subtle regulatory differences in LHPA physiology can only be uncovered when the endogenous LHPA system is dormant and responses to stimuli remain unaffected by endogenous hormonal bursts.

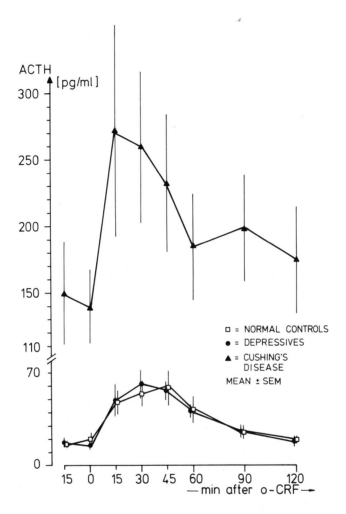

Fig. 7

ACTH release following 100 ug ovine-CRH adminis- tered at 8 am to patients with ACTH-dependent Cushing's disease (n=9), patients with major endo- genous depression (n=8) and normal controls (n=8). From Müller et al. (28) and Holsboer et al. (29).

BEHAVIORAL NONENDOCRINE EFFECTS OF CRH

It has been documented by several investigators that CRH containing neurons and fibers are ubiquitous in the brain suggesting an involve- ment in function other than corticotropin cell regulation and hormone release. The view that CRH is involved in mediation of central nonendocrine effects is supported by recently reported animal studies (34-46) which are summarized in Fig.8.

Collectively, these data allow one to suggest that CRH hyperactivity in the CNS is not only a key factor in mediating stress response but also involved in etiopathology of depression. Since CRH was found to be elevated in the CSF of depressives the conclusions extracted from animal behavior studies may well have clinical implications, where loss of appetite, disturbed sleep, altered autonomous function, psychomotor disturbances, loss of sexual drive and anxiety are yardsticks to diagnose major depression.

We have routinely applied a battery of self-rating scales to normal controls before and after h-CRH challenges without any sign of change. However, we found some alterations of sleep architecture induced by h-CRH when infused shortly before and after falling asleep which suggest that also peripherally administered h-CRH can modulate this behavioral complex (47).

BEHAVIORAL EFFECTS OF CENTRAL CRH

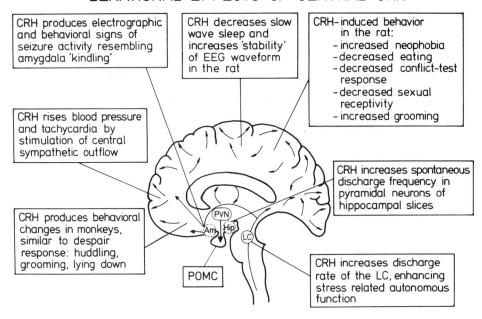

CRH produces electrographic and behavioral signs of seizure activity resembling amygdala 'kindling'

CRH decreases slow wave sleep and increases 'stability' of EEG waveform in the rat

CRH-induced behavior in the rat:
- increased neophobia
- decreased eating
- decreased conflict-test response
- decreased sexual receptivity
- increased grooming

CRH rises blood pressure and tachycardia by stimulation of central sympathetic outflow

CRH increases spontaneous discharge frequency in pyramidal neurons of hippocampal slices

CRH produces behavioral changes in monkeys, similar to despair response: huddling, grooming, lying down

CRH increases discharge rate of the LC, enhancing stress related autonomous function

Fig. 8

Animal studies converge to the postulate that central overactivity of CRH secreting neurons precipitate behavioral changes which resemble depressive behavior in humans.

Effects of h-CRH upon sleep-eeg

Fifty ug h-CRH or placebo were infused to eleven healthy male volunteers (aged 28.3 ±5.9 yrs, range 20-37) four times every hour beginning at 10 pm. All subjects fell asleep after 11 pm. No immediate effects of repetitive h-CRH stimulations during the first part of the night were observed when conventional guidelines for sleep stages are used. However, in the second part of the night high frequency contents increased while at the same time slow wave sleep (stage 3 and 4) became significantly reduced (Tab. 1). Also the percentage of REM sleep decreased following h-CRH whereas REM-density remained unchanged. Importantly, these effects of h-CRH were not associated with significantly increased awakenings, stage shifts, movements, or differences in sleep period times. The observation of a more shallow sleep after repeated h-CRH administration as opposed to placebo suggests that peripheral hormonal overactivity of the pituitary-adrenocortex system contributes to the

Table 1. Effect of h-CRH upon selected sleep characteristics in normal male controls

	h-CRH	Saline	P
1. half of the night			
REM-latency (min)	93.9 ± 10.4	95.3 ± 12.0	NS
REM-amount %	11.4 ± 1.5	11.4 ± 1.3	NS
Stage I/II %	61.8 ± 2.9	55.3 ± 4.4	NS
Stage III/IV %	22.8 ± 2.9	26.4 ± 3.7	NS
2. half of the night			
REM-amount	21.5 ± 2.1	27.1 ± 2.2	0.02
Stage I/II %	63.5 ± 2.3	54.9 ± 2.9	0.01
Stage III/IV %	3.9 ± 0.8	6.0 ± 1.5	0.01

behavioral phenomena which are experimentally and perhaps also physiologically evoked by central CRH. In addition, minute quantities of CRH which may have passed the blood brain barrier can be responsible on the observed effects.

INTERACTION BETWEEN h-CRH INDUCED HORMONAL EFFECTS AND
REGULATION OF THYROTROPIN AND GROWTH HORMONE IN DEPRESSION

Multiple endocrine perturbation tests are considered to provide a set of variables which allow profiling of neural function in depression. This rationale is limited if several neuroendocrine systems depend on each other. We employed h-CRH-tests in combination with other endocrine stimuli in order to investigate whether or not the hypothesis of independent endocrine function is valid.

LHPA-thyroid interaction

Besides abnormality of the pituitary-adrenocortical axis the reduced thyrotropin (TSH) response following infusion of thyrotropin-releasing hormone (TRH) constitutes one of the more extensively studied endocrine disturbance among depressives (48). We compared ACTH response following 100 ug h-CRH with TSH responses to 500 ug TRH in 11 patients with major endogenous depression and 11 normal controls (6). The time difference between both tests was at least two days and basal thyroid status revealed euthyroidism. In agreement with current literature, decreased TSH output expressed as area under time course curves was found in depressives when compared with controls (4.5 ± 3.4 uU x min/ml $\cdot$ 10^2 versus 7.7 ± 3.6 uU x min/ml$\cdot$ 10^2, t = 2.12, df = 20, p$<$ 0.01). A correlation of the net TSH and ACTH output following specific secretagogues revealed statistical significance (r = 0.65; p$<$0.01). In 12 normal controls the pituitary-adrenal axis was challenged during sleep with a total of 200 ug h-CRH during 4 hours (10 pm - 1 am). TRH tests were performed at the next morning which revealed that after h-CRH prestimulation TSH responses to TRH are blunted (Holsboer et al., unpublished observation, Oct. 1985).

It is well accepted that clinical conditions associated with hypercortisolism such as Cushing's disease or exogenous administration of glucocorticoid results in a blunted TSH response after TRH. Also the findings of an association between ACTH and TSH responses after specific stimulation suggests that the thyroid axis is not independent from pituitary-adrenal activity. Both endocrine axes seem to be at last in part under a common control mechanism.

LHPA interaction with growth hormone secretion during sleep

Blunted responses of growth hormone to various pharmacologic probes such as clonidine (49) were reported to occur in depressed patients. On the contrary, the spontaneous secretion of growth hormone during daytime seems to be increased in depression (50). The largest and most consistently timed pituitary release of growth hormone in adults occurs during the first half of the night and this growth hormone surge is regulated in a different mode than during daytime either spontaneously or following pharmacological stimulation (51). In principal, growth hormone is under the influence of two types of peptides with opposite effects: growth hormone releasing factors which stimulate somatotrophic cells at the anterior piuitary level and somatostatin which inhibits growth hormone secretion at the same sites.
We conducted a series of studies in controls and depressives where we sampled blood continuously during sleep and compared hormone secretory patterns with sleep-EEG data.
Whereas growth hormone recordings over the whole night revealed no significant difference between the patients and a matched group of control subjects, the averaged growth hormone values for the depressed patients were significantly lower during the first half of sleeping time (Steiger et al., unpublished observation, May 1986). Interestingly, this difference was independent from any sleep-EEG parameter

including slow wave sleep. This suggests that sleep onset is permissive to both processes, slow wave sleep and growth hormone surge, and that the timely association of both phenomena is rather fortuituous. Since reduced growth hormone output during the first half of the sleep period in depressives was temporally associated with elevated cortisol secretion and increased cortisol nadirs we speculated that the pituitary-adrenal hyperactivity may in part account for a blunted growth hormone release during sleep in depression. This hypothesis was tested in 11 normal male controls, who received intravenous injections of 50 ug h-CRH or saline at 10 pm, 11 pm, 12 pm and 1 am (47). We observed that the cortisol surges induced by h-CRH were associated with a significant blunting of sleep related growth hormone release (see Fig. 9). Because h-CRH probably fails to cross the blood brain barrier to a

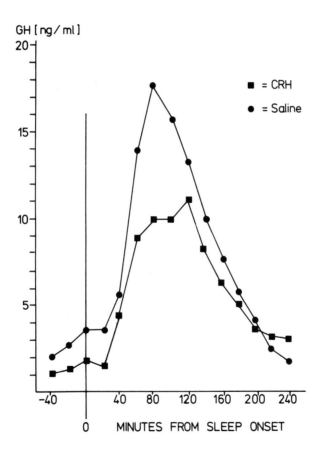

Fig. 9

The area under the time course curve for nocturnal growth hormone (GH) surges during placebo saline infusion was 2.6 ± 0.9 ng x min/ml $\cdot 10^3$ and during h-CRH (50 ug) given at 10 pm, 11 pm, 12 pm and 1 am was 1.2 ± 0.3 ng x min/ml $\cdot 10^3$ (Wilcoxon, $p < 0.01$).

physiologically relevant degree we suspect that enhance cortisol secretion is involved in the observed findings. However, a direct effect of
h-CRH can not be ruled out.

Previous studies by Gillin et al. (52) showed that also ACTH affects
sleep through its action on adrenocortical steroid secretion. They
further documented that the effects depend strongly on the timing of
adrenocortical stimulation. Cortisol secretion during sleep in depression is not only characterized by increased secretion and elevated
nadirs but also by the time of the nocturnal increase of the plasma
cortisol concentration which occurs earlier in relation to EEG-defined
sleep onset (53). Interestingly, during continuous infusion of ovine-
CRH the circadian pattern of cortisol secretion seems to be maintained,
but appeared to be phase advanced. Although all present data are consistent with a mechanism by which hypercortisolism induces blunting of
growth hormone during sleep it needs to be stressed that somatotrophic
cell regulation is extremely complex and a linear relationship between
any particular stimuli and the amount of growth hormone release is
questionable.

COMMENT

Psychoneuroendocrine study of the LHPA-system in patients with depression has yieled convincing evidence that altered hormonal secretion in
a subset of these patients is functionally related to central brain
areas. Major support for this view stems from two findings: (1) Blunted
ACTH response after h-CRH in depression indicates integrity between
pituitary and adrenocortex; and (2) following dexamethasone pretreatment only depressives, but not controls respond with increased ACTH and
cortisol release after stimulation with h-CRH. This points to altered
function of suprapituitary limbic structures most likely at the hippocampus which is a major site for corticosteroid action and also a
structure implicated in processing of learning and memory. This concept
supports that while measuring peripheral hypercortisolism we are in
fact dealing with a centrally induced phenomenon.

Also psychopathological research receives new impetus from such a
strategy since focussing upon the hippocampus as one specifically
affected brain area allows application of tests which examine cognitive
function. Preliminary data from our group (Heuser et al., unpublished
observation, July 1986) and others (54) showed an association between
altered LHPA activation and cognitive function. At present it is unclear, whether LHPA-axis activation and cognitive impairment are
downstream effects of a central disturbance. Alternatively, LHPA-overactivity may impair glucocorticoid receptor containing neurons, resulting in loss of cells which are involved in cognitive function. While
the exact clinical implications of steroid induced effects upon the
limbic system are not fully understood it is obvious that altered
endocrine homeostasis has profound effects upon central neurotransmitter and -receptor function via an afferent limb. It is noteworthy that
glucocorticoid induced effects upon the brain are widespread and not
entirely restricted to the hippocampus, although this area has the
greatest ability to retain glucocorticoids (55) and is the locus where
most of the neurochemical effects of adrenal steroids have been observed. Among these neurochemical effects are changes in ß-adrenergic
receptor binding (56, 57) and suppression of high affinity GABA uptake
by hippocampal synaptosomes (58). The latter finding is of particular

interest, because Majewska et al. (59) recently reported that specific corticosteroid metabolites may amplify the inhibitory effect of GABA upon nerve cell activity.

Recently, the field of psychoneuroimmunology experienced an extraordinary reupsurge. Of particular interest for psychoneuroendocrine research is the role of hormones in CNS-immunological interactions. It is well known, that the immune system is under influence of central processes by means of the neuroendocrine network. The thymus gland is not only under neural and endocrine control but produces substances which are capable to stimulate pituitary corticotrophs. In addition, lymphocytes produce peptides such as interleukin I which also stimulates ACTH release from the pitutiary. On the other hand, each leucocyte is capable to express POMC related products if challenged with CRH in vitro for one or two days (60). Thus, each leucocyte may function as minuscule pituitary corticotroph cell. Collectively, these more recent observations suggest that the LHPA-system acts as a bidirectional link between CNS and immunoendocrine circuits. It is well established that immune systems and endocrine function can be influenced by behavior. Now there is good evidence that behavior and immunoendocrine systems communicate on a two-way track, because, for example, patients hospitalized for severe depression have an impaired immune response (61). Such a reciprocal interaction may take place via the LHPA-system which is frequently overactive in depression. As a preliminary conclusion we submit that in psychopathology associated with LHPA activation one needs to consider altered immune function as one additional source for any observed changes.

Clinical psychoneuroendocrinologists have extensively studied possibilities of comparing altered hormonal function with psychopathological features in order to elaborate biological markers for clinical syndromes or diagnostic attributions. However, such a dualism between function and behavior is probably misleading. We rather suggest, that endocrine or other physiological changes are just another possible mode of expressing behavior. This view gets support from animal studies which demonstrate that immune response (62) or adrenocortical activity (63) can be conditioned. As a consequence altered physiological function such as LHPA pathophysiology in depression could be regarded as a symptomatic, behavioral feature ready to be incorporated in diagnostic schedules which use multiaxial descriptions.

Depression represents a complex of diseases which share several common features but have a variety of causes. Recent studies employing h-CRH have extended our knowledge of pathophysiology which underlies hypercortisolism in a subset of depressed patients. Additionally, behavioral studies in animals provided evidence that also nonendocrine effects of LHPA-hormones are involved in precipitation and symptomatology of depression. Within such a framework the biopotency of h-CRH in central structures is likely to be involved in the expression of affective disorder and may play a key role in mediating the observed effects. However, it would be premature to submit that CRH tests will finally resolve etiopathology of human depression.

REFERENCES

1. Vale, W., Spiess, J., Rivier, C., Rivier, J. (1981): Science, 213: 1341-1397.
2. Shibahara, S., Morimoto, Y., Furutani, Y., Notake, M., Takahashi H., Shimizu, S., Horikawa, S., Numa, S. (1983): The EMBO J., 2: 775-779.
3. Schulte, H.M., Chrousos, G.P., Booth, J.D., Oldfield, E.H., Gold, P.W., Cutler, G.B. jr., Loriaux, D.L. (1984): J. Clin. Encorinol. Metabol., 58: 192-196.
4. Schürmeyer, T.H., Augerinos, P.C., Gold, P.W., Gallucci, W.T., Tomai, T.P., Cutler, G.B. jr, Loriaux, D.L., Chrousos, G.P. (1984): J. Clin. Endocrinol. Metab., 59: 1103-1108.
5. Holsboer, F., von Bardeleben, U., Gerken, A., Stalla, G.K., Müller, O.A. (1984): The New Engl. J. Med., 311: 1127.
6. Holsboer, F., Gerken, A., von Bardeleben, U., Grimm, W., Beyer, H., Müller, O.A., Stalla, G.K. (1986): Biol. Psychiat., 21: 601-611.
7. Spitzer, R.L., Endicott, J., Robins, E. (1978): New York State Psychiat. Inst. , New York.
8. Gold, P.W., Chrousos, G.P., Kellner, C., Post, R., Roy, A., Augerinos, P., Schulte, H., Oldfield, E., Loriaux, L. (1984): Amer. J. Psychiat., 141: 619-627.
9. Gold, P.W., Loriaux, D.,L., Roy, A., Kling, M.A., Calabrese, J.R., Kellner, C.H., Nieman, L.K., Post, R.M., Pickar, D., Gallucci, W., Augerinos, P., Paul, S., Oldfield, E.H., Cutler, G.B.jr., Chrousos, G.P. (1086): The New Engl.J. Med., 314: 1329-1335.
10. Holsboer, F., Gerken, A., Stalla, G.K., Müller, O.A. (1987): Amer. J. Psychiat., 144: 229-231.
11. Hullin, R.P., Levell, M.J., O'Brien, M.J., Toumba, K.J. (1981): Brit. J. Psychiat., 138: 373-380.
12. Holsboer, F., Doerr, H.G., Sippell, W.G. (1982): Psychoneuroendocrinol., 7: 155-162.
13. Hermus, A.R.M.M., Pieters, G.F.F.F., Smals, A.G.H., Benraad, T.J., Kloppenborg, P.W.C. (1984): J. Clin. Endocrinol. Metab., 58: 187-191.
14. Reul, J.M.H.M., de Kloet, E.R. (1985): Endocrinol., 117: 2505-2511.
15. von Bardeleben, U., Holsboer, F., Stalla, G.K., Müller, O.A. (1985): Life Sciences, 37: 1613-1618.
16. Holsboer, F., von Bardeleben, U., Wiedemann, K., Müller, O.A., Stalla, G.K. (1987): Biol. Psychiat., 22: 228-234.
17. Nemeroff, G.B., Widerlöv, E., Bissette, G., Walleus, H., Karlsson, I., Eklund, K., Kilts, C.D., Loosen, P.T., Vale, W. (1984): Science 226: 1342-1344.
18. Holsboer, F., Wiedemann, K., Boll, E. (1986): Arch. Gen. Psychiat., 43: 813-815.
19. Tornello, S., Ortis, E., De Nicola, A.F., Rainbow, T.C., McEwen, B.S. (1982): Neuroendocrinol., 35: 411-417.
20. Sapolsky, R.M., Krey, L.C., McEwen, B.S. (1984a): Endocrinol., 114: 287-292.
21. Sapolsky, R.M., Krey, L.C., McEwen, B.S. (1984b): Procl. Nat. Acad. Sci. USA, 81: 6174-6177.
22. Serby, M., Richardson, S.B., Rypma, B., Twente, S., Rotrosen, J.P. (1986): Biol. Psychiat., 21: 971-974.
23. Rubinow, D.R., Post, R.M., Gold, P.W., Ballenger, J.C., Reichlin, S. (1985): Psychopharmacol., 85: 210-213.

24. Holsboer, F. (1983): Pharmacopsychiat., 16: 186–191.
25. Rees, L.H., Besser, G.M. (1977): Lancet, i: 726–728.
26. McIntyre, I.M., Oxenkrug, G.F. (1984): Biol. Psychiat., 19: 1725–1729.
27. Dave, J.R., Eiden, l.E., Karanian, J.W., Eskay, R.L. (1986): Endocrinol., 118: 280–286.
28. Müller, O.A., Hartwimmer, J., Hauer, A., Kaliebe, T., Schopohl, J., Stalla, G.K., von Werder, K. (1986): Psychoneuroendocrinol., 11: 49–60.
29. Holsboer, F., Müller, O.A., Doerr, H.G., Sippell, W.G., Stalla, G.K., Gerken, A., Steiger, A., Boll, E., Benkert, O. (1984): Psychoneuroendocrinol., 9: 147–160.
30. Van Cauter, E., Refetoff, S. (1985): The New Engl. J. Med., 312: 1343–1349.
31. Holsboer, F., von Bardeleben, U., Gerken, A. (1986): In: New Results in Depression Research, edited by Hippius, H., Klerman, G., and Matussek, N., pp. 217–249. Springer Verlag, Berlin, Heidelberg, New York, Tokyo.
32. Holsboer, F., Gerken, A., Steiger, A., Benkert, O., Müller, O.A., Stalla, G.K. (1984): The Lancet, i: 55.
33. Holsboer, F., Gerken, A., Stalla, G.K., Müller, O.A. (1985): Biol. Psychiat., 20: 276–286.
34. Koob, G.F., Bloom, F.E. (1985): Federation Proc., 44: 259–263.
35. Sutton, R.E., Koob, G.F., Le Moal, M., Rivier, J., Vale, W. (1982): Nature, 297: 331–333.
36. Thatcher-Britton, K., Morgan, J., Rivier, J., Vale, W., Koob, G.F. (1985): Psychopharmacol., 86: 170–174.
37. Britton, D.R., Koob, G.F., Rivier, J., Vale, W. (1982): Life Sci., 31: 363–367.
38. Britton, D.R., Varela, M., Garcia, A., Rosenthal, M. (1986): Life Sci., 38: 211–216.
39. Brown, M.R., Fisher, L.A. (1985): Federation Proc., 44: 243–248.
40. Smythe, G.A., Grunstein, H.S., Bradshaw, J.E., Nicholson, M.V., Compton, P.J. (1984): Nature 308: 65–67.
41. Sirinathsinghji, D.J.S., Rees, L.H., Rivier, J., Vale, W. (1983): Nature 305: 232–235.
42. Rivier, C., Rivier, J., Vale, W. (1986): Science 231: 607–609.
43. Kalin, N.H. (1986): Biol. Psychiat., 21: 124–140.
44. Kalin, N.H. (1985): Federation Proc., 44: 249–253.
45. Ehlers, C.L., Reed, T.K., Henriksen, S.J. (1986): Neuroendocrinol., 42: 467–474.
46. Aldenhoff, J.B., Gruol, D.L., Rivier, J., Vale, W., Siggins, G.R. (1983): Science, 221: 875–877.
47. Holsboer, F., von Bardeleben, U., Benkert, O., Herth, T., Hiller, W., Nehring, K., Steiger, A., Stein, A. (1986), In: Biological Psychiatry 1985, edited by Shagass, C. et al., pp. 150–152. Elsevier, New York, Amsterdam, Tokyo.
48. Loosen, P.J., Prange, A.R.jr. (1982): Amer. J. Psychiat., 139: 405–416.
49. Matussek, N., Ackenheil, M., Höhe, M., Müller-Spahn, F. (1986): In: Biological Psychiatry 1985, edited by Shagass, C. et al., pp. 788–790. Elsevier, New York, Amsterdam, Tokyo.
50. Mendlewicz, J., Linkowsky, P., Kerkhofs, M., Desmedt, D., Golstein, J., Copinschi, G., van Cauter, E. (1985): J. Clin. Endocrinol. Metab., 60: 505–512.

51. Mendelson, W.B., Jacobs, L.S., Gillin, J.C., Wyatt, R.J. (1979): Psychoneuroendocrinol., 4: 341–349.
52. Gillin, J.C., Jacobs, L.S., Snyder, S., Henkin, R.I. (1974): Neuroendocrinol., 15: 21–31.
53. Jarrett, D.B., Coble, P.A., Kupfer, D.J. (1983): Arch. Gen. Psychiat., 40: 506–511.
54. Rubinow, D.R., Post, R.M., Savard, R., Gold, P.W. (1984): Arch. Gen. Psychiat., 41: 279–283.
55. Mc Ewen, B.S. (1982): In: Current Topics in Neuroendocrinology, edited by Ganten, D., and Pfaff, D., pp. 1–22. Springer, Berlin, Heidelberg, New York, Tokyo.
56. Mobley, P.L., Sulser, F. (1980): Nature, 286: 608–609.
57. Roberts, D.C.S., Bloom, F.E. (1981): Europ. J. Pharmacol., 74: 37–41.
58. Miller, A.L., Chaptal, C., Mc Ewen, B.S., Pech, E. (1978): Psychoneuroendocrinol., 3: 155–164.
59. Majewska, M.D., Harrison, N.L., Schwartz, R.D., Barker, J.L., Paul, S.M. (1986): Science, 232: 1004–1007.
60. Smith, E.M., Morrill, A.C., Meyer, W.J.III, Blalock, J.E. (1986): Nature, 321: 881–882.
61. Schleifer, S.J., Keller, S.E., Meyerson, A.T., Raskin, M.J., Davis, K.L., Stein, M. (1985): Arch. Gen. Psychiat., 41: 484–486.
62. Ader, R., Cohen, N., Bovbjerg, D. (1982): J. Comp. Physiol. Psychol., 96: 517–521.
63. Levine, S., Cooper, G.D. (1976): Physiol. Behav., 17: 35–37.

The Hypothalamic-Pituitary-Adrenal Axis:
Physiology, Pathophysiology, and Psychiatric
Implications, edited by A.F. Schatzberg and
C.B. Nemeroff. Raven Press, Ltd., New York
© 1988.

THE RELEVANCE OF CORTICOTROPIN RELEASING HORMONE TO NORMAL PHYSIOLOGY AND TO PATHOPHYSIOLOGIC ALTERATIONS IN HYPOTHALAMIC-PITUITARY ADRENAL FUNCTION

Philip W. Gold, M.D.[1], Harvey J. Whitfield, M.D.[1],
Mitchel A. Kling, M.D.[1], Mark A. Demitrack, M.D.[1],
Harry A. Brandt, M.D.[2], and George P. Chrousos, M.D.[3]

[1]Biological Psychiatry Branch, National Institute of Mental
Health, Bethesda, MD 20892
[2]Laboratory of Clinical Science, National Institute of
Mental Health, Bethesda, MD 20892
[3]Developmental Endocrinology Branch, National Institute of
Child Health and Human Development, Bethesda, MD 20892

INTRODUCTION

The first definitive demonstration of hypothalamic influence upon anterior pituitary function came in 1955, when Saffron and Schally showed that hypothalamic fragments possessed corticotropin releasing properties when incubated with pituicytes in vitro (40). This discovery validated a prediction made by the eminent physiologist Geoffrey Harris seven years earlier (21). Although pituitary responsiveness to the hypothalamus was first demonstrated via a corticotropin releasing factor, the sequencing of corticotropin releasing hormone (CRH) by Vale, et al., came only in 1981 (54), years after the amino acid sequence of a number of other hypothalamic hormones had already been elucidated (e.g. TRH, SRIF, LH-RH). A number of reasons account for the delay in the sequencing of CRH. First, in contrast to hypothalamic hormones such as TRH, which is a tripeptide, or LH-RH, which is a decapeptide, the structure of CRH is much more complex, consisting of 41 amino acids (54). Moreover, its biologic potency can be virtually abolished by oxidation or by deletion of even a small component of its overall sequence. This vulnerability of CRH to oxidation and the requirement for most of the 41 amino acid sequence for full biologic activity probably reflects to necessity for careful regulation of a hormone whose functional activity is required for survival.

The monumental work by Vale et al. in sequencing CRH was first accomplished in the sheep (54). Shortly thereafter, Rivier isolated a similar, but not identical, 41 amino acid CRH in the rat (rCRH) (33). Later, Numa's group sequenced the genes of both ovine CRH (oCRH) and human CRH (hCRH) and deduced the amino acid sequence of the corresponding peptides (13,49). Surprisingly, both the rCRH and the hCRH appeared to be chemically identical. Moreover, both oCRH and hCRH are structurally similar, each containing 41 amino acids and showing 83% homology.

The sequencing and subsequent synthesis of CRH has greatly enhanced our capacity to explore the hypothalamic-pituitary-adrenal axis in the normal "resting" state and during stress. Also, it has allowed us to study the hypothalamic-pituitary components of Cushing's disease and adrenal insufficiency and has enhanced our capacity to evaluate psychiatric conditions associated with hypercortisolism. Such states include depression (9,39), anorexia nervosa (14), alcoholism (51), and obsessive-compulsive neurosis (23). On occasion the hypercortisolism seen in depressive illness and alcoholism can be so severe that it is difficult to distinguish them from Cushing's disease; hence each of these psychiatric entities has been referred to by some endocrinologists as a "pseudo-Cushing's state."

Of interest is that CRH is synthesized not only by the hypothalamus for transport by hypophyseal portal blood but, like other hypothalamic hormones such as TRH and somatostatin, is distributed and/or synthesized in many other brain regions (5,12,27), and like these peptides seems to play a role in coordinating complex physiological and/or behavioral processes. Specifically, it has been shown that there are extensive aggregations of CRH cell bodies and terminal fields in the limbic system, cortex, and in close association with the central autonomic system and the locus ceruleus (5,12,27). This distribution of CRH within and beyond the hypothalamus provides an anatomical context for the observation that CRH can simultaneously activate and coordinate metabolic (7), circulatory (7), and behavioral responses that are adaptive in stressful situations (6,50,52). Hence, in the rat, intracerebroventricular (ICV) administration of CRH leads not only to activation of the HPA axis but also to activation of the sympathetic nervous system (7) and to several behavioral changes characteristic of the stress response, including decreased feeding (6) and sexual behavior (50), and assumption of a freeze posture in a foreign environment (52). In addition, ICV CRH causes a marked increase in hostility when administered in familiar surroundings and induces limbic seizures which show cross-sensitization with electrically kindled seizures (57).

Given CRH's significant role in HPA regulation and its intriguing effects on CNS function, we embarked on a series of clinical studies with CRH in normal volunteers and in patients with endocrine disturbances characterized by abnormal hypothalamic-pituitary-adrenal function, including Cushing's syndrome, adrenal insufficiency, and in psychiatric patients with major psychiatric disorders characterized by hypercortisolism. In volunteers, we hoped to examine the physiological relevance of CRH to pituitary-adrenal function in man as well as to explore the differential biological effects and pharmacokinetics of oCRH and hCRH under varying conditions. In our patient populations, we asked the following questions: (1) Can CRH help determine whether the hypercortisolism in depression reflects an alteration in the setpoint for feedback inhibition of cortisol on ACTH secretion at a pituitary locus, versus the possibility of an alteration in the secretion of endogenous CRH; (2) Can CRH help in the differential diagnosis of the various hypercortisolemic syndromes; (3) Can CRH be helpful in the differential diagnosis of Cushing's syndrome and adrenal insufficiency; and (4) Is CRH of possible relevance to the overall symptom complex of major psychiatric illnesses such as depression and anorexia nervosa?

Studies with CRH in Normal Volunteers

We first studied normal controls to compare naturalistically occurring ACTH pulses to those induced by hCRH administration. Our data showed that spontaneous endogenous ACTH and cortisol pulses (isolated during circadian sampling) closely resembled those induced by an intra-venous bolus of 1 ug/kg of hCRH (2,24,43). This finding led to an addi-tional experiment designed to further explore the relationship between pulsatile CRH secretion and the pattern of ACTH and cortisol secretion in the basal state. In this study we asked the following questions: Could hCRH, given in pulses to simulate the temporal distribution of expected, naturally occurring ACTH secretory episodes restore the func-tion of the pituitary-adrenal axis seen in patients with CRH deficien-cy (i.e., secondary adrenal insufficiency due to corticotroph-sparing [suprapituitary] lesions) (3). Human CRH was given as a 1 ug/kg bolus eight times during a 24-hour period. The timing of each pulse of hCRH was chosen to correspond to the expected times of ACTH pulsation under naturalistic conditions based on our circadian studies in normal vol-unteers. Hence, the majority of the pulses were given in the early morning hours to correspond with the a.m. cortisol surge. To a degree which was unexpected, such a paradigm of hCRH pulsatile administration reproduced the normal amplitude and circadian variation of cortisol secretion in patients with hypothalamic-CRH deficiency (3).

We had previously noted that a continuous infusion of oCRH in nor-mal volunteers for 24 hours produces a pattern of cortisol secretion which includes preservation of its circadian rhythm; though the ampli-tude is blunted compared to that of the naturalistic rhythm induced by the hCRH pulses (44). Thus, although basal circadian cortisol secre-tion may be dependent on endogenous CRH secretion, this circadian pat-tern of pituitary-adrenal function may also involve a component of a circadian rhythm in the responsiveness to CRH itself (44). Preliminary results from frequent CSF sampling of human subjects indicate that CSF CRH concentrations have a circadian rhythm which is inverse to that of plasma cortisol (unpublished information).

In addition to studies of the relevance of CRH to basal and circa-dian ACTH and cortisol secretion, we have also attempted to assess the relationship of CRH to pituitary-adrenal function during stress. To accomplish this task, we have attempted to see whether the ACTH respon-ses to frequent pulses of hCRH given at 30 to 90 minute intervals from 1800 to 2000h would produce an ACTH secretory pattern resembling that seen during the standard insulin tolerance test or during strenuous exercise. We noted that ACTH and cortisol responses to repeated pulses of hCRH were much less than those seen during the insulin tolerance test (3) or during strenuous exercise (24). Although neutralization of endogenous CRH in rats by administration of anti-CRH antibodies abol-ishes more than 75% of the ACTH responses to insulin-induced hypogly-cemic stress (34), our data are compatible with previous suggestions that factors other than CRH play an important role in producing the ACTH responses seen during stress. Putative factors which may under-lie these extra-CRH influences on stress-induced ACTH secretion include the catecholamines and arginine vasopressin (7), both of which are known to increase during hypoglycemia and other forms of stress (4,29,33). In support of the possible role of vasopressin are our recent data obtained in normal volunteers which shows that osmotically-induced vasopressin secretion potentiates CRH-induced ACTH secretion, compatible with other studies showing synergism between exogenous vasopressin administration and CRH in human volunteers (32). We doubt that oxytocin participates in CRH-induced ACTH secretion, despite a suggestion from in vitro stu-dies, where it has been shown to have synergy with CRH in causing ACTH secretion.

In an additional stress-related study (24), we examined the effects of treadmill exercise at three different exercise intensities (50, 70, and 90% VO_2 max) to find an intensity-dependent activation of the pituitary-adrenal axis with no activation occurring at 50%. Studies of joggers running less than 40 miles/wk and obligate athletes running over 40 miles/wk showed that the dose-response between the activation of the pituitary-adrenal axis and the absolute amount of workload or O_2 consumption was shifted to the right in proportion to the degree of training. These results suggest that athletes can produce the same amount of work with much less activation of their hypothalamic-pituitary-adrenal axis.

Development of a Clinically Applicable CRH Stimulation Test

To ascertain the clinical applications of CRH, we initiated a series of studies in volunteers to assess the following questions: (1) Which peptide (oCRH or hCRH) might be best to use in acute challenges of the pituitary-adrenal axis; (2) What dose should be administered in these studies and for how long should hormonal responses be sampled; (3) What time of day would be best suited for the performance of dynamic stimulation of the human pituitary-adrenal axis? To assess these questions we conducted pharmacokinetic and dose-response studies with both oCRH and hCRH.

The first dose response study with oCRH in primates was performed by our group in cynomolgus macaques (46). Corresponding studies in man yielding similar results were performed by Orth et al. (28). These studies show that the lowest maximal stimulatory dose for cortisol secretion was 1 ug/kg; moreover, this dose produced clearcut plasma cortisol and ACTH secretion in all volunteers and experimental animals without detectable adverse effects. Of particular interest was the fact that the ACTH and cortisol responses to oCRH were prolonged, remaining clearly elevated at the end of the three-hour sampling period (28,46).

In our similar dose-response studies with hCRH in nonhuman primates (43) and man (42), Schuermeyer et al. noted a dose-dependent increase of plasma ACTH and cortisol concentrations with greater doses of hCRH. Peak plasma ACTH and cortisol responses to hCRH were significantly lower than those achieved by oCRH (43,42). Moreover, the ACTH and cortisol responses to hCRH were of much briefer duration than those with oCRH. Accordingly, comparisons of the time-integrated secretory responses of both ACTH and cortisol following hCRH administration indicate that oCRH is several times more potent than hCRH (43,42). This difference is mainly due to the longer-lasting effect of oCRH upon ACTH and cortisol secretion.

These longer-lasting effects of oCRH on ACTH and cortisol secretion can be presumably accounted for on the basis of the differences in pharmacokinetic properties of oCRH (45) and hCRH (42,43,). Hence, in our study directly comparing the metabolic clearance rate of these two peptides in human volunteers, Schuermeyer et al. noted that hCRH is cleared from plasma much more rapidly than oCRH. On the basis of thes data hCRH seemed more suitable than oCRH for studies of pulsatile ACTH secretion, whereas oCRH appeared suitable for studying patients.

An additional factor of relevance to the establishment of a clinically applicable CRH stimulation test was the determination of an optimal time of day for administration of the peptide to patient populations. To explore this question, we administered a 1 ug/kg bolus of oCRH at 9 a.m., near the time of day when the axis is most active, and at 8 a.m., when the axis is normally quiescent. It was found that owing to the lower baseline cortisol levels seen in the evening, the net integrated cortisol responses to oCRH are greater at this time (47). Hence, we decided that our CRH stimulation test would consist of the 1 ug/kg bolus of oCRH given at 8 p.m.

Studies in Psychiatric Illnesses Characterized by Hypercortisolism

Patients with Depression

The first major finding utilizing CRH in psychiatry was made by our group when we noted that drug-free depressed patients showed a significantly blunted ACTH response to oCRH (17). This was followed by a report by Holsboer et al. using hCRH (22). The finding of an attenuated response to oCRH in depression suggested that the pituitary corticotroph cell in depressed patients was appropriately restrained by the negative feedback effects of elevated cortisol levels (16,17) This was supported by a significant negative correlation between basal cortisol levels and the ACTH response to CRH in depression (16,17). In light of the apparently "normal" corticotroph cell function in depressed patients, we first advanced the hypothesis that hypercortisolism in depression represents a defect at or above the hypothalamus which results in the hypersecretion of endogenous CRH. To test this hypothesis, we attempted to replicate in normal controls a situation in which the pituitary corticotroph cell is exposed to excessive corticotropin releasing hormone. In order to accomplish this, we administered a continuous infusion for 24 hours and evaluated the ACTH and cortisol responses (44). Of interest is the fact that the circadian rhythm of cortisol is preserved despite the continuous administration of oCRH, suggesting that the pituitary corticotroph cell shows a diurnal sensitivity to exogenous CRH. This is of interest in light of the fact that the circadian rhythm of cortisol is also generally preserved in depression (20). Of additional interest is the fact that the mean amplitude of cortisol secretion during continuous CRH infusion is elevated about 40% to 50%, and that the urinary-free cortisol secretion during CRH infusion averaged 150 to 200 ug/day (44). Hence, the amplitude of plasma cortisol during the 24-hour period and the magnitude of urinary-free cortisol hypersecretion is very similar during conditions of continuous administration of oCRH to controls and in the endogenously depressed state. We concluded, therefore, that a continuous CRH infusion to normal volunteers reproduces the pattern and magnitude of hypercortisolism typically associated with depression. Additional data compatible with the idea that CRH is hypersecreted in depressed patients derives from the data of Nemeroff et al. who showed that the level of CSF CRH is elevated in depression (28). Although we could not demonstrate a significant elevation of CSF CRH in depressed patients, these subjects did manifest a significant positive correlation between post-dexamethasone cortisol levels in depressed patients and the CSF level of CRH (36). Moreover, we noted that CSF CRH is significantly higher in depressed patients who are dexamethasone non-suppressors than in dexamethasone suppressors.

Inspection of our ACTH and cortisol responses to CRH in depression revealed other salient features of HPA dysfunction in depressed patients. For instance, we noted that depressed patients showed robust total and free cortisol response despite the very small ACTH released during CRH stimulation (16,17). We surmise from these data that the adrenal cortex in depression has grown hyperresponsive to ACTH (16,17), compatible with the well-described phenomenon of progressive functional and anatomical hypertrophy of the adrenal cortex seen during either experimentally induced stress (48) or during the course of chronic and repeated hyperstimulation of the adrenal cortex by ACTH in man (31). This suggestion of adrenal hyperresponsiveness to ACTH in depression is compatible with the data of Amsterdam et al. who showed that chronically depressed patients manifest greater cortisol responses to a bolus of exogenous ACTH than normal subjects (1).

Although our depressed patients were hypercortisolemic, it is noteworthy that basal ACTH levels were only slightly elevated (16,17). This rather modest increase in plasma ACTH levels in depression most likely reflects a normal corticotroph cell caught in the balance between forces (i.e., negative feedback exerted by a hyperactive adrenal cortex from below and a predominating excess of CRH drive from above). Hence, the corticotroph cell, though restrained by the negative feedback to secrete at a rate that produces only slightly elevated ACTH levels, is nevertheless sufficiently driven by CRH to promote excessive cortisol secretion by hyperplastic adrenals. Presumably, depressed patients would have shown elevated levels of ACTH in the beginning of their depressive illness.

Whether CRH plays a role in any human disease apart from the rare cases of Addison's disease secondary to CRH deficiency and the rare cases of ectopic CRH secretion remains to be established. Its possible involvement in depression, however, is intriguing in light of the following four sets of findings taken from the disciplines of developmental psychology, clinical psychiatry, and neurophysiology (17): 1.) Laboratory animals subjected to maternal deprivation during the neonatal period show significant hyperactivity of the hypothalamic-pituitary adrenal axis during stress throughout adult life (53). Hence such animals presumably show a permanent change in the responsivity of their CRH neuron; 2.) Individuals who are depression-prone are thought to show greater than usual incidence of early noxious stress or maternal deprivation. Clinical experience shows that such a history seems to produce a tendency to repetitively relive the intense anxiety and dysphoria associated with this early deprivation throughout adult life whenever a significant frustration or important loss occurs. Thus, such individuals also seem prone to hyperresponsivity of their CRH neuron intermittently throughout life; 3.) CRH given ICV to animals not only stimulates the hypothalamic-pituitary-adrenal axis (35) but also activates the locus ceruleus (56), produces decreased eating (6) and sexual behavior (50), and causes significant changes in activity (52); 4.) CRH has been reported to induce limbic seizures which cross-sensitize with electrically kindled seizures (57). These findings, taken together, suggest that a CRH model of depression could help integrate dynamic formulations which take into account early losses and subsequent internal and external stress as factors which can predispose to or precipitate major depression, and the observations that depressed subjects often show hypercortisolism, significant anxiety, anorexia, diminished libido, hypo- or hyperactivity, and respond at times to limbic anticonvulsants (30). That changes in CRH may be related to depressive symptomatology is also supported by empirical observations that depression is perhaps the only major symptom represented in a substan-

volunteers suggests that CRH may be involved in both exercise and lactate-induced panic. Hence both the pituitary-adrenal and lactate responses correlated positively with each other and with the magnitude of exercise stress; moreover, in concentrations achieved during moderate and strenuous exercise, we have shown that lactate produces a dose-dependent increase in the in vitro release of CRH from rat hypothalami (unpublished observations). An additional finding suggesting a role for CRH in the panic disorder syndrome is our finding that alprazolam produces a dose-dependent decrease in pituitary-adrenal function in unrestrained primates and inhibits the CRH response to serotonin in our in vitro rat hypothalamic organ culture system. Parenthetically, the effect of alprazolam on these parameters was significantly greater than that of diazepam, compatible with its greater efficacy in both panic disorder and depression.

Differential Diagnosis of Cushing's Syndrome

Cushing's syndrome as a spontaneous pathophysiological entity can be divided into three types: Cushing's syndrome due to pituitary hypersecretion of ACTH (Cushing's disease), hypercortisolism secondary to ectopic secretion of ACTH, and the autonomous secretion of cortisol by an adrenal adenoma or carcinoma. Thus, Cushing's syndrome can be divided into ACTH-dependent (the pituitary and ectopic CTH secretion syndromes) and ACTH-independent (the cortisol producing adrenal neoplasms) subsets. The differential diagnosis between the two types of ACTH-dependent Cushing's syndrome is often difficult. In contrast, adrenal tumors are usually diagnosed radiologically or by ultrasound. The most sensitive procedure for this diagnosis is high resolution computerized axial tomography or magnetic resonance imaging of the adrenal glands.

We and others have shown that the CRH stimulation test appears to differentiate between Cushing's disease and the ectopic ACTH syndrome (10,11). Thus, whereas most patients with Cushing's disease show exaggerated to robust ACTH responses to CRH, patients with the ectopic ACTH syndrome generally fail to respond to CRH. Comparison of this test with the standard low dose-high dose dexamethasone suppression test shows that the former is equal or better (26). Considering that the CRH test is a two-hour outpatient procedure, there are many advantages in including it in our differential diagnosis testing. We have also shown that CRH testing in Cushing's syndrome can be done in the morning without losing its diagnostic power.

Patients with ACTH-independent Cushing's syndrome had undetectable levels of plasma ACTH throughout the test and their plasma cortisol concentrations remained unlatered, like the patients with ectopic ACTH secretion. Medical or surgical correction of the hypercortisolism was followed quickly by normalization of the CRH response (10,11).

Differential Diagnosis of Adrenal Insufficiency

Adrenal insufficiency is divided pathophysiologically into two types: primary, when the adrenals are primarily responsible, and secondary, when either the pituitary gland or the hypothalamus fails. We administered CRH to patients with adrenal insufficiency to determine whether the CRH stimulation test would be useful in the differential diagnosis of this condition (47).

Patients with primary adrenal failure had high basal plasma ACTH levels and low basal cortisol values. Cortisol levels were low or undetectable throughout the test. Plasma ACTH values were markedly stimulated by CRH. Similarly, patients with secondary adrenal insufficiency also had low or undetectable basal levels of cortisol and cortisol responses to CRH were generally absent or minimal. However, in contrast to the group with primary adrenal insufficiency, though basal plasma ACTH concentrations were low in these subjects, the plasma ACTH responses to CRH were variable. Some patients had no ACTH responses to a CRH bolus, in contast to the majority of patients who showed an early ACTH response similar to normal subjects. The response of many of these latter subjects, however, did not plateau but continued to increase during the test. We postulate that the patients who showed no ACTH response to CRH represent corticotroph cell failure (pituitary adrenal insufficiency); on the other hand, the patients who responded to CRH have endogenous CRH insufficiency or inability of hypothalamic CRH to reach the pituitary (hypothalamic adrenal insufficiency). We conclude from these data that, in contrast to the experience with other hypothalamic releasing factors such as LHRH and TRH, CRH may differentiate pituitary from hypothalamic causes of secondary adrenal insufficiency without a need for priming by multiple releasing hormone injections.

Two patients with the rare syndrome of acquired idiopathic isolated ACTH deficiency had adrenal insufficiency with adrenocorticol responses to a 48-hour ACTH stimulation test characteristic of the secondary form. These subjects also failed to respond to insulin-induced hypoglycemia and to vasopressin. These patients had undetectable plasma ACTH and cortisol responses to a bolus of CRH. Thus, they appeared to have pituitary rather than hypothalamic adrenal insufficiency.

Cushing's Disease vs. Depression

Patients with Cushing's disese often show signs of clinical depression. Conversely, the hypercortisolism of depression can be of sufficient magnitude that it has been termed a pseudo-Cushing's state. Although there has been controversy over the years concerning the etiology of the hypercortisolism associated with Cushing's disease and affective illness, the overlap in the clinical and biochemical manifestations of these illnesses has prompted some to suggest that they share common pathophysiological features. Of clinical significance is the fact that patients with primary depression who may be hirsute or obese and who manifest high plasma and urinary-free cortisol levels can be impossible to distinguish from patients with mild or early Cushing's disease preceding the physical stigmata such as the buffalo hump or purple striae by months or even years.

Data from our group and others show that despite profound basal hypercortisolism, patients with Cushing's disease generally show hyperresponsiveness of the pituitary corticotroph cell to exogenous CRH. Thus, in contrast to patients with depression who show a pituitary corticotroph cell normally responsive to the negative feedback effects of glucocorticoids, patients with Cushing's disease manifest a pituitary corticotroph cell which is grossly unresponsive to cortisol negative feedback effects.

Our data also suggest that the differences in pituitary corticotroph cell function between depressed and Cushing's disease patients seems accompanied by differences in hypothalamic CRH neuron function. Specifically, we have shown that many of our patients with Cushing's disease whom we studied one week after selective transsphenoidal adenomectomy (at a time when basal ACTH and crotisol were uniformly undetectable) showed normal or nearly normal plasma ACTH responses to exogenous CRH (11). We surmise that the adrenal insufficiency in each of these post-operative patients reflects hypofunction of corticotropin releasing factor neurons which had been physiologically suppressed by exposure to the negative feedback of their long-standing hypercortisolism. This formulation is supported by our recent finding that compared to depressed patients and controls, CSF CRH concentration is significantly lower in Cushing's disease patients (unpublished data).

The differential pathophysiology of hypercortisolism which we propose for Cushing's disease and depression is manifested by the fact that responses to CRH in these disorders are in the opposite direction (e.g., an exaggerated ACTH response in Cushing's diesase and a blunted one in depression). In all other diagnostic tests which have been utilized to differentiate depression from Cushing's disease, such as the dexamethasone suppression test and serial urinary-free cortisol determinations, responses and/or levels in depression and Cushing's disease have been in the same direction. Thus, the CRH stimulation test could assist in the differential diagnosis between depression and early Cushing's disease. Indeed, our data show that the CRH stimulation test is helpful in the differential diagnosis of these disorders, with about 25% of Cushing's disease patients showing ACTH responses to CRH in the depressed patient range and vice versa (16).

SUMMARY

The isolation of CRH has provided an unparalleled opportunity for study of the central component of pituitary-adrenal function. Moreover, the finding that the ICV administration of CRH can coordinate a complex series of behavioral and physiological responses adaptive during stressful situations has made the study of this peptide of even greater interest to investigators attempting to explore fundamental pathophysiological mechanisms in patients with psychiatric illnesses characterized at some time during their course by hypercortisolism.

Over the past five years our group has attempted to explore the physiological relevance of CRH to human pituitary-adrenal function and to develop strategies to employ either the administration or the measurement of this peptide in clinical studies. After advancing several lines of indirect evidence which indicated that CRH played an important role in the pulsatile secretion of the pituitary corticotroph cell, we concluded that hCRH could be helpful in studying the dynamics of corticotroph cell function while oCRH (which we showed functioned as a long-acting analog of hCRH) would be most suitable for a CRH stimulation test applied for diagnostic purposes.

The application of this CRH stimulation test, in concert with measurement of CRH in the CSF, has helped to elucidate the pathophysiology of hypercortisolism in depression, anorexia nervosa, and panic disorder. Hence, blunted ACTH responses to oCRH in these disorders indicated that the pituitary corticotroph cell was appropriately restrained by basal hypercortisolism, indicating a defect at or above the hypothalamus resulting in the hypersecretion of endogenous CRH. In support of this hypothesis was the finding in anorexia nervosa patients of frankly elevated CSF CRH levels and in depressed patients of CSF CRH levels which correlated positively with the degree of pituitary-adrenal activation. In addition, a continuous infusion of CRH to volunteers produced hypercortisolism whose pattern and magnitude closely resembled that seen in depression.

Our studies with CRH have also helped to elucidate the pathophysiology of hypercortisolism in Cushing's disease and to settle the controversy regarding whether depression and Cushing's disease represent similar or distinct pathophysiological entities. Hence, in contrast to depressed patients exaggerated ACTH responses to oCRH in Cushing's disease patients (despite pronounced hypercortisolism) indicated that the pituitary corticotroph cell in Cushing's disease subjects is grossly unresponsive to glucocorticoid negative feedback. Moreover, in contrast to depressed patients, whose hypothalamic CRH neuron seemed hyperfunctional despite hypercortisolism, the CRH neuron in patients with Cushing's disease seemed appropriately suppressed by long-standing hypercortisolism. This differential pathophysiology between depression and Cushing's disease constitutes the basis for the utility of the CRH stimulation test in the often difficult differential diagnosis posed by these two disorders.

Whether CRH plays a critical role in the symptom complex of major psychiatric disorders characterized by hypercortisolism remains a question which can only be answered by further pre-clinical and clinical investigation. Additional elucidation of the regulation of the hypothalamic CRH neuron and its relationship to the CNS CRH system should help in the development of pharmacologic approaches aimed at suppressing the CRH system. Conceivably, such agents could be therapeutic adjuncts in the treatment of depression and related disorders. Ultimately the development of CRH antagonists which can gain access to the central nervous system after their peripheral administration may be required to more fully evaluate the role of CRH in major psychiatric illness.

REFERENCES

1. Amsterdam, J. D., Winokur, A., Abelman, E., Jucki, I., and Rickels, K. (1983): Am. J. Psychiatry, 140:907-909.
2. Avgerinos, P. C., Schuermeyer, T. H., Gold, P. W., Nieman, L., Udelsman, R., Loriaux, D. L., and Chrousos, G. P. In: Hormones and Pulsatility, edited by W. Growley, (in press), Plenum Press, New York.
3. Avgerinos, P. C., Schuermeyer, T. H., Gold, P. W., Tomai, T. P., Loriaus, D. L., Sherins, R. J., Cutler, G. P., Jr., and Chrousos, G. P. (1986): J. Clin. Endocrinol. Metab., 62:816-821.
4. Axelrod, J. and Reisine, T. D. (1984): Science, 22:452-459.
5. Bloom, F. E., Battenberg, E. L. F., Rivier, J., and Vale, W. (1982): Regul. Pept., 4:43-48.
6. Britton, D. R., Koob, G. F., and Rivier, J. (1982): Life Sci., 31: 363-367.
7. Brown, M. R., Fisher, L. A., Spiess, J., Rivier, C., Rivier, J., and Vale, W. (1982): Endocrinology, 111:928-931.
8. Cantwell, D. P., Sturzengerger, S., and Burnough, J. (1977): Arch. Gen. Psychiatry, 34:1087-1094.
9. Carroll, B. J., Curtis, G. C., and Mendels, J. (1976): Arch. Gen. Psychiatry, 33:1039-1044.

10. Chrousos, G. P., Nieman, L., Nisula, B., Schulte, H. M., Gold, P. W., Cutler, G. B., Jr., and Loriaux, D. L. (1984): New Engl. J. Med., 311:472-473.
11. Chrousos, G. P., Schulte, H. M., Oldfield, E. H., Gold, P. W., Cutler, G. B., and Loriaux, D. L. (1984): New Engl. J. Med., 310:622-627.
12. De Souza, E. B., Perrin, H. M., Insel, T., Rivier, J., Vale, W., and Kuhar, M. J. (1984): Science, 224:1449-1450.
13. Furatani, Y., Morimoto, Y., Shubahara, S., Noda, M., Takahashi, H., Hirose, T., Asai, M., Inayama, S., Hayashida, H., Miyata, T., and Numa, S. (1983): Nature, 301:537-540.
14. Gerner, G. H. and Gwirtsman, H. E. (1981): Am. J. Psychiatry, 138:650-653.
15. Gillies, G. E., Lingo, E. A., and Lowry, P. J. (1982): Nature, 299:355-357.
16. Gold, P. W., Loriaux, D. L., Ropy, A., Kling, M. A., Calabrese, J. R., Kellner, C. H., Post, R. M., Pikar, D., Gallucci, W. T., Avgerinos, P. C., Paul, S., Oldfield, E. H., Cutler, G. B., and Chrousos, G. P. (1986): N. Engl. J. Med. 314:1329-1335.
17. Gold, P. W., Chrousos, G. P., Kellner, C. H., Post, R. M., Roy, A., Avgerinos, P. C., Schulte, H. M., Oldfield, E. H., and Loriaux, D. L. (1984): Am. J. Psychiatry, 141:619-627.
18. Gold, P. W., Gwirtsman, H., Avgerinos, P. C., Nieman L., Gallucci, W. T., Kaye, W., Jimerson, D., Ebert, M., Rittmaster, R. W., Loriaux, D. L., and Chrousos, G. P. (1986): New Engl. J. Med. 314:1335-1342.
19. Guillemin, R., Vargo, T., Rossier, J., Minick, S., Ling, N., Rivier, C., Vale, W., and Bloom, F. (1977): Science, 197:13671368.
20. Halbreich, V., Asnis, G. M., Slindledecker, R., Zumoff, B., and Nathan, R. S. (1985): Arch. Gen. Psychiat. 42:909-915.
21. Harris, G. W. (1948): Physiol. Rev., 28:134-179.
22. Holsboer, F., Genken, H., Stalla, G. K., Muller, G. H. (Letter) (1984): New Engl. J. Med., 311:1127.
23. Insel, T. R., Kalin, W. H., Guttmacher, L. B., Cohen, R. M., and Murphy, D. L. (1982): Psychiatrty Res., 6:153-160.
24. Luger, A., Deuster, P., Kyle, S. B., Montgomery, L. C., Gallucci, W. T., Gold, P. W., Loriaux, D. L., and Chrousos, G. P. (1986): Clin. Res. 34:421.
25. Nemeroff, C. B., Widerlov, E., Bissette, G., Wallens, H., Karllson, I., Edlund, K., Kilts, G., and Loosen, P. (1984): Science, 224: 1342-1344.
26. Nieman, L. K., Chrousos, G. P., Oldfield, E. H., Avgerinos, P. C., Cutler, G. B., Jr., and Loriaux, D. L. (1986): Ann. Int. Med. (in press).
27. Olschowska, J. A., O'Donohue, T. L., Mueller, G. P., and Jacobowitz, D. M. (1982): Peptides, 3:995-1015.
28. Orth, D. N., Jackson, R. V., DeCherney, G. S., Debold, C. R., Alexander, A. N., Island, D. P., Rivier, J., Rivier, C., Spiess, J., and Vale, W. (1983): J. Clin. Invest., 71: 587-595.
29. Plotsky, P. M., Rubin, T. O. and Vale, W. (1985): Endocrinology, 117:323-329.
30. Post, R. M. (1982): Psychol. Med., 123:70-104.
31. Renoud, A. E., Jenkins, D., and Thorn, G. W. (1952): J. Clin. Endocrinol. Metab., 12:763-797.

32. Rittmaster, R., Cutler, G. B., Jr., Brandon, D., Gold, P. W., Loriaux, D. L., and Chrousos, G. P. (1986): Clin. Res. 34:432.
33. Rivier, J., Spiess, J., and Vale, W. (1983): Proc. Natl. Acad. Sci. USA, 80:4851-4855.
34. Rivier, C. and Vale, W. (1983): Nature, 35:325-327.
35. Rock, J. P., Oldfield, E. H., Schulte, H. M., Chrousos, G. P., Gold, P. W., Cutler, G. B., Jr., Kornblith, P. L., Loriaux, D. L., and Chrousos, G. P. (1984): Brain Res., 323:365-368.
36. Roy, A., Pickar, D., Chrousos, G. P., Doran, A., Paul, S. M., Loriaux, D. L., and Gold, P. W.: Am. J. Psychiatry (in press).
37. Roy, A., Pickar, D., Doran, A., Paul, S. M., Chrousos, G. P., and Gold, P. W.: Am. J. Psychiatry (in press).
38. Roy-Byrne, P. P., Uhde, T., Post, R. M., Gallucci, W. T., Chrousos, G. P., and Gold, P. W.: Am. J. Psychiatry (in press).
39. Sachar, E. J., Hellman, L., Fukushima, D. K. and Gallagher, T. F. (1970): Arch. Gen. Psychiatry, 23:289-298.
40. Saffran, M., Schally, A. V., and Bentey, B. G. (1955): Endocrinology, 57:439-444.
41. Schally, A. V., Chang, R. C., Arimura, A., Redding, T. W., Fishback, J. B., and Vigh, S. (1981): Proc. Natl. Acad. Sci. USA, 78:5197-5201.
42. Schuermeyer, T. H., Avgerinos, P. C., Gold, P. W., Tomai, T. P., Gallucci, W. T., Cutler, G. B., Jr., Loriaux, D. L., and Chrousos, G. P. (1984): J. Clin. Endocrinol. Metab., 59:1103-1108.
43. Schuermeyer, T. H., Gold, P. W., Gallucci, W. T., Tomai, T. P., Cutler, G. B., Jr., Loriaux, D. L., and Chrousos, G. P. (1985): Endocrinology, 117:300-306.
44. Schulte, H. M., Chrousos, G. P., Gold, P. W., Booth, J. P., Oldfield, T. H., Cutler, G. B., Jr., and Loriaux, D. L. (1985): J. Clin. Invest. 75:1781-1785.
45. Schulte, H. M., Chrousos, G. P., Gold, G. W., Oldfield, E. H., Phillips, J. M., Munson, P. J., Cutler, G. B., Jr., and Loriaux, D. L. (1982): J. Clin. Endocrinol. Metab., 55:1023-1027.
46. Schulte, H. M., Chrousos, G. P., Oldfield, E. H., Gold, P. W., Cutler, G. B., Jr., and Loriaux, D. L. (1982): J. Clin. Endocrinol. Metab., 55:810-812.
47. Schulte, H. M., Chrousos, G. P., Oldfield, E. H., Gold, P. W., Cutler, G. B., Jr., and Loriaux, D. L. (1985): Horm. Res. 21:69-74.
48. Selye, H. (1936): Nature (London), 138:32.
49. Shibahara, S., Morimoto, Y., Furatani, Y., Notake, M., Takahashi, H., Shimizu, S., Horikawa, S., and Numa, S. (1983): The EMBO J., 2:775-779.
50. Sirinathsinghji, D. J. S., Rees, L. H., Rivier, J., and Vale, W. (1983): Nature, 305:232-235.
51. Stokes, P. E. (1973): Ann. N. Y. Acad. Sci., 215:77-81.
52. Sutton, R. E., Koob, G. F., Le Moal, M., Rivier, J., and Vale, W. (1982): Nature, 297:331-333.
53. Thomas, E. B., Levine, E. S., and Arnold, W. J. (1968): Dev. Psychobiol., 1:21-23.
54. Vale, W., Spiess, J., River, C., and Rivier, J. (1981): Science, 213:1394-1397.
55. Vale, W., Vaughn, J., Smith, M., Yamamoto, G., River, J., and Rivier, C. (1983): Endocrinology, 113:1121-1131.
56. Valentino, R., Foote, S. L., and Aston-Jones, G. (1983): Brain Res., 220:363-367.

57. Weiss, S. R. B., Post, R. M., Gold, P. W., Chrousos, G. P., and Pert, A. (1986): Brain Res., 372:345–351.
58. Yates, A., Leehey, K., and Shisslak, C. M. (1983): N. Engl. J. Med., 308:251–255.

The Hypothalamic-Pituitary-Adrenal Axis: Physiology, Pathophysiology, and Psychiatric Implications, edited by A.F. Schatzberg and C.B. Nemeroff. Raven Press, Ltd., New York © 1988.

WHAT IS THE RELATIONSHIP BETWEEN PLASMA ACTH AND PLASMA

CORTISOL IN NORMAL HUMANS AND DEPRESSED PATIENTS?

K. Ranga Rama Krishnan, M.D., James C. Ritchie, M.P.H.,
Ananth N. Manepalli, M.D., Sanjeev Venkataraman, M.D.
Randal D. France, M.D., Charles B. Nemeroff, M.D., Ph.D.
and Bernard J. Carroll, M.D., Ph.D.

Duke University Medical Center, Box 3215
Durham, North Carolina   27710

INTRODUCTION

In the thirty years following the discovery of antide-pressant drugs considerable research has been conducted on the pathophysiology of depressive illness. One of the methods used to study this question has been the neuroendo-crine strategy. This strategy has been based on the assump-tion that dysfunction in the limbic system or other extra-hypothalamic brain areas (believed to be areas involved in the pathophysiology of affective disorders) may be reflected by alterations in neuroendocrine function. This hypothesis is rendered plausible by the finding that cer-tain of the limbic system areas such as the amygdala and hippocampus in addition to their involvement in normal and abnormal behavioral states also regulate neuroendocrine function.

The neuroendocrine axis which has been studied in the greatest detail in patients with mood disorders is the hypothalamic-pituitary-adrenal (HPA) system. Early studies demonstrated increased 17-hydroxy-corticosteroid secretion in depressed patients compared to normals [5,34,35]. This led to further research demonstrating other abnormalities in the HPA axis in depression. These abnormalities include a phase advance in cortisol secretion [46], inability to suppress cortisol secretion by dexamethasone [46], increased frequency of pulsatile peaks of cortisol, (more so in the evening than in the daytime) and blunting of the ACTH response to CRF [17]. However, very little is actu-ally known about the pathophysiology of these abnormalities of the HPA system in depression.

As noted above, one of the classic assumptions has been that these HPA axis abnormalities reflect changes in limbic system activity. To demonstrate that this assumption might be true, it must be clearly shown that the increased corti-

sol secretion is secondary to increased adrenocortico-
trophin (ACTH) secretion from the anterior pituitary and
that this, in turn, is secondary to increased secretion of
corticotropin-releasing factor (CRF) (or other peptides
like vasopressin with CRF-like activity) from the hypothalamus. Finally all of these changes must ultimately be
shown to be due to altered limbic system activity.

Although for a number of years ACTH was considered the
sole agent regulating cortisol release from the adrenal,
there is now evidence that this view may be an oversimpli-
fication. Early studies of 24 hour cortisol and ACTH
secretion patterns in normal subjects by Krieger et al [25]
suggested that there were periods when there was a dissociation between cortisol and ACTH secretion, but these
investigators considered these findings to be anomalous
episodes [25]. On closer reexamination of their data, it
is seen that rather than being anomalous, such episodes
were quite frequent. Further, there was very little corre-
lative relationship between ACTH and cortisol secretion.
This might have been due to a variety of factors including
assay methodology, timing of collection and processing of
the samples. More recent work by Fehm et al [10] suggests
that dissociation of cortisol and ACTH secretion is not
uncommon. This group first showed that methamphetamine
administration produced an increase in cortisol secretion
without a significant change in ACTH secretion [10]. However, the assay which they used was not a very sensitive
one and this raised an important question, namely did
increased cortisol secretion occur in these studies with
changes in ACTH secretion that were physiologically significant, but below the detection threshold of their assay.
In addition Fehm et al [11] showed that the early morning
secretion of cortisol often is not preceded by any significant change in ACTH secretion. Again, this study used the
same, relatively insensitive ACTH assay.

In a third study, Fehm et al [12] examined the secretion
of cortisol following an afternoon meal. They demonstrated
that the post-prandial rise in plasma cortisol concentrations was not accompanied by a significant rise in ACTH
secretion. On the basis of these three studies, Fehm et al
[10] postulated the existence of factors other than ACTH
that play a physiological a role in cortisol secretion.
They also suggested the possibility of direct or indirect
sympathetic activation of adrenocortical secretion.

Our research group recently began a series of studies
in order to determine whether there is a dissociation of
ACTH and cortisol secretion in normal individuals and in
depressed patients.

METHOD

Normal volunteers with no current or past psychiatric
history were recruited by advertisement. Depressed
patients admitted to the Affective Disorders Unit at Duke
University Medical Center were entered in the study if

they met inclusion criteria. All patients admitted to the study were drug free for at least seven days. They were medically healthy on the basis of a physical examination and routine laboratory examination. None of the patients met any of the exclusion criteria listed by Carroll for the Dexamethasone Suppression Test [4]. All patients admitted to the study met Research Diagnostic Criteria [41] for major depressive disorder, endogenous subtype. The diagnosis was determined on the basis of a structured SADS (Schedule for Affective Disorders and Schizophrenia) interview [8]. On day 1 of the study an intravenous catheter was placed in the antecubital vein at 2130 h. Serial blood samples were collected for measurement of plasma ACTH and cortisol throughout the night. Between 2230 h and 0100 h, blood was collected at 30 minute intervals and between 0100 h and 0800 h at 15 minute intervals. On the following day subjects received 1 mg of dexamethasone orally at 2300 h. Blood for measurement of plasma ACTH and cortisol were collected at 0800 h, 1600 h and 2200 h the following day. We used a highly sensitive radioimmunoassay for ACTH with a sensitivity of less than 1 pg/ml. The primary antiserum for this assay was produced in our laboratory by immunizing New Zealand White female rabbits, with a thyroglobulin conjugate of ACTH 11-24. This fragment was chosen to maximize the epitope of the antiserum with the bioactivity (steroidogenic activity) of ACTH 1 to 39 and to reduce cross-reactivity with other pro-opiomelanocortin (POMC) derived peptides. Only ACTH 11-24, 18-29 (CLIP) and 1-24 exhibit any significant cross-reactivity. The epitope of the antiserum appears to be in the 18-24 region of the ACTH molecule. Blood samples for this assay are placed in EDTA-containing vacutainer tubes (chilled on ice). Within ten minutes the blood is centrifuged at 1200 g for ten minutes at 2° C. to separate the plasma. The plasma is harvested, the volume is measured and 0.2 ml of 1.0N of HCL is added for every 1.0 ml of plasma. The plasma is then frozen at -80° C. until extraction, never longer than five days.

Plasma exhibits high non specific interaction with this assay system, probably as a result of interference with antigen-antibody binding by MR type plasma proteins. To overcome this problem the plasma is extracted by using C 18 Sep-pak cartridges (Waters Associates, Milford, Massachusetts). The frozen acidified plasma is thawed and centrifuged at 6200 g for ten minutes at 2° C. The pH must be less than 2.0. The plasma sample is then applied to a Sep-pak cartridge which has been pretreated with methanol, 8M urea, and water. After the sample is bound to the cartridge, the cartridge is rinsed with water and 4% acetic acid. The ACTH is eluted from the Sep-pak with 4ml of 4% acetic acid in 90% ethanol. The samples are then dried in a speed rack concentrator (Savant Instruments, Farmingdale, NY). The dry extracts are stored at -80° C until assay. Using this extraction technique, recovery of radiolabeled ACTH averages 80 to 90% (using 125 I -ACTH).

Although we have been able to show no difference

between standard curves prepared in ACTH stripped plasma
(ASP) and those prepared in assay vehicle, standards are
routinely prepared in ASP and processed through the Sep-pak
procedure.   This guarantees that the samples and standards
are identical, thus negating matrix effects and alleviating
the necessity for recovery corrections.

Due to its concentrating nature, when enough sample is
available, the extraction procedure also allows us to
improve the sensitivity of the assay into the 0.2 to 0.5
pg/ml range. On the day of assay, the dried extracts and
standards are dissolved in freshly made 0.1% recrystallized
human albumin (Schwartz/Mann, Spring Valley, NY) in water
(assay vehicle).   The pH of this solution has been previously adjusted to 3.6 using 1.0N hydrochloric acid. Each
assay tube contains 250 μl of standard sample assay
vehicle and 100 ul of primary antiserum at a 1:80,000 dilution in assay buffer.   The final dilution is 1:600,000.
The assay buffer is as follows: 0.055 M sodium phosphate
buffer, 0.02% sodium azide, 0.02% poly-L-lysine, 1.25% normal rabbit serum and 0.5% Triton X-100, pH 7.40.   All
pipetting and sample handling is done on ice. The tubes
are mixed and held at 4° C. for 18 hours. One hundred ul
of ^{125}I-ACTH, dissolved in assay buffer is added to each
tube. This represents approximately 4,000 CPM and 5 pg of
ACTH. The tubes are again mixed and held at 4° C. for five
hours. Second antibody, goat anti-rabbit gamma globulin,
(Arnel Products, New York, NY) is then added. The tubes
are again mixed and maintained at 4° C for 1 hour. Two mls
of deionized H_2O are then added to each tube and they are
centrifuged at 6,000 g for 20 minutes at 2° C.   The tubes
are decanted and the pellets are counted in a Multi-Prias
gamma counter (Packard Instruments, Downer's Grove, Ill.).
The 80, 50 and 20% B/Bo points have averaged 5.6, 24.4, and
127.7 fmol/ml respectively (1 fmol/ml=4.51 pg/ml).   The
standard curve is run from 0.7 to 177 fmol/ml in quadrupli-
cate and the sensitivity of the assay for 1 ml of plasma is
1 pg/ml.   The interassay C.V. is 12% and the intra-assay
C.V. is 7% at a level of 5.6 fmol/ml.

The assay has been validated using plasma from hypophysectomized humans (all values undetectable) and plasma
obtained during insulin tolerance tests (peak values 3 to 6
times baseline values). In normal subjects baseline values
range from 0.89 to 11.08 fmol/ml in the morning and from
0.22 to 6.7 fmol/ml in the evening. Morning values after
one mg of dexamethasone overnight in normal subjects range
from 0.22 to 6 fmol/ml. As further validation, pooled
human plasma has been tested with this antiserum immobi-
lized on an affinity column matrix. Over 95% of the material bound to the antiserum was ACTH$_{1-39}$. Comparison of
our ACTH assay and that of Dr. David Orth of Vanderbilt
University yielded a correlation of .9313 for 7 samples
over the concentration range 0.89 to 11 fmol/ml. Cortisol
was measured by a competitive protein binding method.   The
details of this method have been previously described [33].

RESULTS

Preliminary results from the four patients with depression and the first four normal volunteers are illustrated. Figure I shows the night time secretion of cortisol and ACTH in a normal volunteer. Low plasma concentrations of cortisol and ACTH are seen basically throughout the night. Cortisol begins to peak only in the morning and is not preceeded by a significant ACTH peak. Figure II illustrates the night time and early morning secretion of cortisol and ACTH in another normal subject. Again, there is evidence of dissociation between plasma cortisol and ACTH concentrations. There is a significant increase in ACTH without any significant change in cortisol at 0230 hours. Figure III illustrates the night time ACTH and cortisol secretion in a third normal volunteer. In this volunteer there seems to be a clear increase in plasma cortisol concentrations preceded by a rise in plasma ACTH levels. Figure IV illustrates the secretion pattern in a fourth subject. In this subject for one episode there is significant correlation between cortisol increase and ACTH change. In another episode there is no correlation between the two. Similar patterns of dissociation have been observed in other normal volunteers. However some normal volunteers, like subject III, exhibit a clear association between ACTH and cortisol secretion. Approximately 40% of volunteers have grossly disassociated patterns of secretion.

Figure V shows the night time cortisol and ACTH secretion patterns in a depressed individual. This patient had an early morning surge in cortisol secretion and in addition, increased plasma cortisol concentrations throughout the night. These high concentrations are accompanied by significant increases in plasma ACTH concentration only towards the end of the night. Figure VI shows the results obtained in a severely depressed patient with melancholic features. Hypersecretion of cortisol occurs throughout the night. However plasma ACTH concentrations remained low throughout the night with almost no fluctuation. Figure VII shows the cortisol and ACTH secretion patterns in a depressed patient. This patient's plasma cortisol surge commences earlier than usual, between 2 and 4 a.m. Cortisol secretion at this time is not accompanied by ACTH secretion, though cortisol secretion later on in the night is accompanied by ACTH peaks. Figure VIII shows plasma cortisol and ACTH secretion in another depressed patient. In this individual there is an association between cortisol and ACTH secretion in the early morning, but there is no association between ACTH secretion and the cortisol peak which occurs at about 0400 hours. Similar results have been obtained in several other depressed patients.

DISCUSSION

Our data strongly suggest that the assumption that cortisol secretion is <u>alway</u> regulated by changes in ACTH con-

FIGURE I

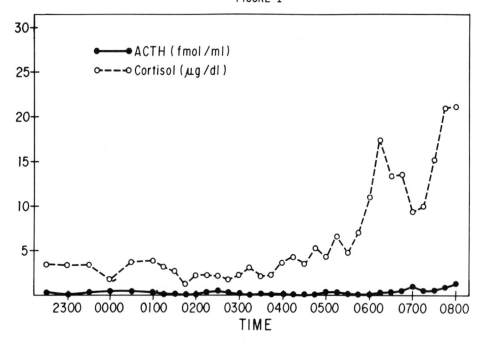

FIGURE II

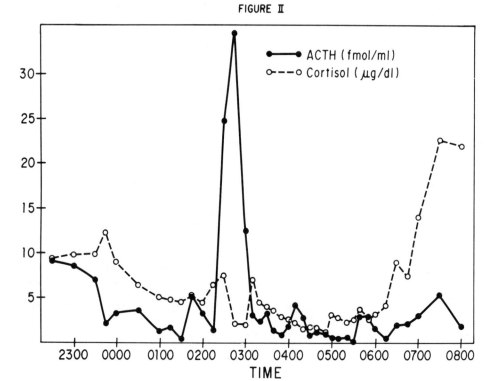

Figures I & II — NOCTURNAL AND EARLY MORNING PLASMA ACTH AND CORTISOL
SECRETION IN NORMAL SUBJECTS.

FIGURE III

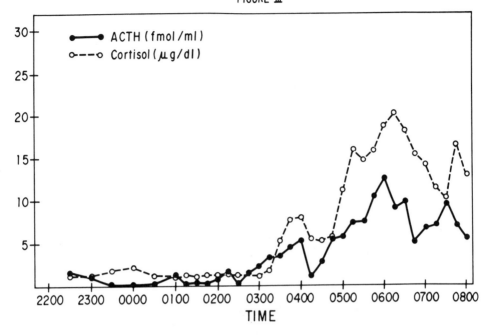

FIGURE IV

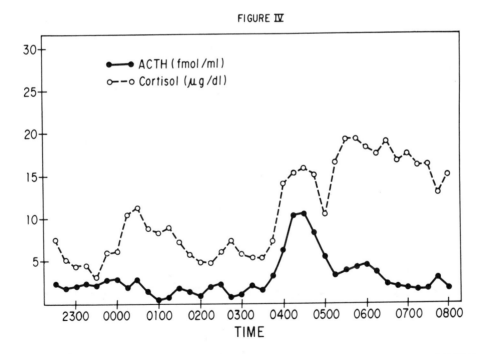

Figures III & IV - NOCTURNAL AND EARLY MORNING PLASMA ACTH AND CORTISOL
SECRETION IN NORMAL SUBJECTS.

FIGURE V

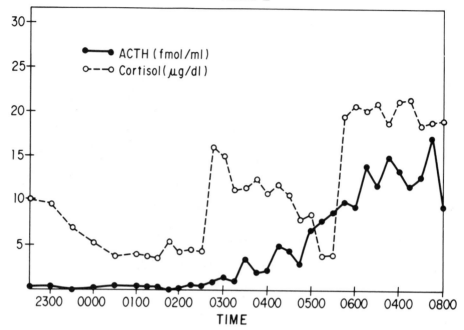

FIGURE VI

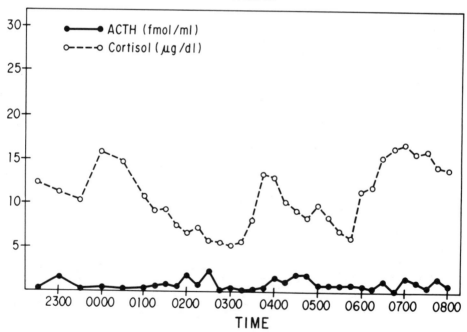

Figure V & VI – NOCTURNAL AND EARLY MORNING PLASMA ACTH AND CORTISOL
SECRETION IN DEPRESSED PATIENTS.

FIGURE VII

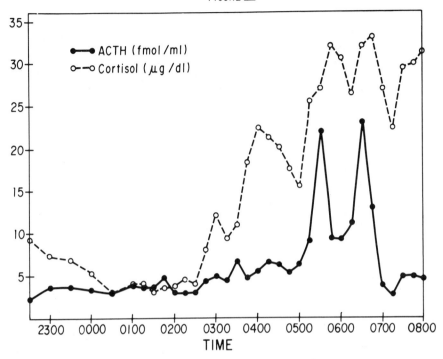

FIGURE VIII

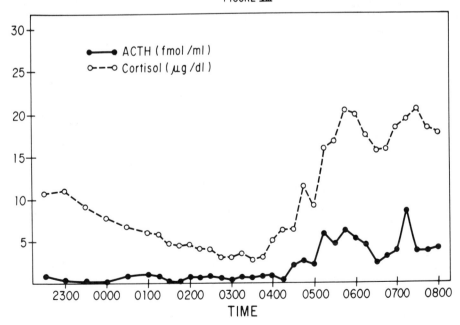

Figure VII & VIII - NOCTURNAL AND EARLY MORNING PLASMA ACTH AND CORTISOL
SECRETION IN DEPRESSED PATIENTS.

centration is incorrect. We have also shown that depressed
individuals generally appear to hypersecrete cortisol in
the earlier part of the night as well as exhibit a phase
advance of the early morning cortisol peak. The results
replicate previous findings of Fehm et al [10] showing similar patterns of dissociation between cortisol and ACTH
secretion in normals. The results also replicate those of
Sherman et al [39] showing similar patterns of dissociation
between cortisol and ACTH in depressed patients.

What is the non-ACTH mechanism?

The short answer is, nobody knows. Three possibilities
are emerging in the current literature: (1) direct sympathetic innervation of the adrenal cortex; (2) indirect sympathetic activation of the adrenal cortex by a paracrine
intermediate step involving the adrenal medulla; (3)
humoral factors that modulate adrenal responsiveness to
ACTH or directly stimulate the adrenal.

Direct Innervation

Forty years ago Marthe Vogt reported increased adrenocortical secretion in dogs after stimulation of the spanchnic
nerve and after close arterial injection of acetylcholine
into the adrenal gland [45]. In 1951 Kiss reported that the
adrenal medulla of the dog and cat receives preganglionic
sympathetic fibers from ventral roots T_{7-9} while the
adrenal cortex receives postganglionic fibers from the spinal ganglia T_{9-11} [21]. Garcia-Alvarez confirmed a sympathetic innervation of the human adrenal cortex and Unsicker
described the electron microscopic appearance of efferent
and afferent sympathetic fibers in the rat and pig adrenal
cortex [15,44]. He summarized evidence for an autonomic
influence on the cortex, including the unilateral changes
in the zona fasciculata produced by unilateral circumscribed hypothalamic lesions [15]. Neostigmine or physos-
tigmine can release corticosterone in hypophysectomized
rats and the daily rhythm of adrenocortical sensitivity to
ACTH also may be mediated by cholinergic innervation of the
adrenal cortex [22,23]. Taken together, these observations
make a prima facie case for considering sympathetic innervation of the adrenal cortex as one possible mechanism of
the non-ACTH extra-pituitary secretion of cortisol. Human
data relevant to this idea come from a study of severe
stress in patients with head injuries. These patients
often fail to suppress cortisol even after doses of 30-60
mg dexamethasone per day [13]. Raised intracranial pressure with an intact brain stem is required for this to
occur, increased intracranial pressure alone being insuffi-
cient. The inference is that the descending sympathetic
pathways through the brain stem mediate the cortisol secretion after a very high dose of dexamethasone in such
patients.

Paracrine Mechanism

Modulation of adrenomedullary PNMT enzyme activity and epinephrine synthesis by glucocorticoids from the adrenal cortex is well established [2]. The reverse possibility, modulation of adrenocortical activity by products of the adrenal medulla, is less well founded, but recently other peptides have been found in the human adrenal medulla. These peptides include several fragments of POMC, including ACTH [9,28,42]. It is possible that if ACTH were released in such close proximity to the adrenal cortex, its target organ, one may expect pronounced effects on blood steroid levels. The adrenal medulla has further been shown to contain enkephalins, CRF, neurotensin and vasoactive-intestinal peptide [16,30]. Interesting support for this hypothesis is provided by a case report [37]. Schteingart et al studied a 41 year old woman with Cushing's Syndrome who had an adrenal medullary tumor and marked adrenocortical hyperplasia. Her hypercortisolism was unaffected by dexamethasone, metyrapone or ACTH. Selective venous catheterization showed that the tumor was the source of ACTH and that the increased cortisol secretion occurred due to hyperplasia of the adrenal cortex. The tumor was found to contain large amounts of ACTH.

If paracrine activation of the cortex from the medulla does occur, then it may be associated with neurally stimulated release of epinephrine. Association of epinephrine and cortisol secretion would then be predicted. Conversely, if direct sympathetic innervation activates the cortex, then this may be reflected in generalized sympathetic activation and the association of norepinephrine and cortisol secretion would be predicted. In principle, therefore, plasma epinephrine or norepinephrine secretion linked with non-pituitary ACTH mediated cortisol secretion could distinguish these two putative mechanisms because, in general, plasma epinephrine changes reflect adrenomedullary activation while plasma norepinephrine changes reflect generalized sympathetic activation.

Another possibility is suggested by the work of Soliman who has shown that the circadian rhythm of glucocorticoids persists in hypophysectomized rats pretreated with ACTH [40]. Administration of a phenylethanolamine N-methyl transferase (PNMT) inhibitor which inhibits epinephrine synthesis abolished the diurnal fluctuation of plasma cortisol. Adrenal enucleation achieved the same effect. Administration of epinephrine restored the rhythm. Addition of an acetylcholinesterase inhibitor increased circulating cortisol. On the basis of this work it is possible to hypothesize that parasympathetic activation of the adrenal medulla with release of epinephrine may play some role in the regulation of cortisol secretion from the adrenal cortex. If this was the case, plasma epinephrine may or may not be related to cortisol secretion but may need to be present in sufficient quantities for cortisol fluctuations to occur.

Humoral Factors

The adrenal cortex contains receptors for a number of hormones besides ACTH and several of these may be capable of modulating the adrenocortical secretion. These include growth hormone, alpha-melanocyte stimulating hormone (alpha-MSH), interferons, prostaglandins and other peptides derived from the thymus and the thyroid gland which have not been fully characterized.

Gamma$_3$-MSH: ACTH is a cleavage product of the prohormone, POMC. The n-terminal region of this peptide designated as the 16 K fragment includes melanotropin (alpha-MSH) and gamma$_3$-MSH. Pedersen et al [31] synthesized a peptide containing gamma$_3$MSH and showed that this peptide stimulates the activity of cholesterol ester hydrolase in the adrenal cortex and potentiates ACTH stimulation of corticosterone release in the hypophysectomized rat. Gamma$_3$-MSH, in contrast to ACTH, did not have any effect on cholesterol side chain cleavage activity. ACTH did not have any effect on cholesterol ester hydrolase. Thus the effect was shown to be qualitatively different. Gamma$_3$-MSH has been shown to be present in the circulation of several species including humans [38]. The physiological importance of this peptide has been suggested by the work of Sharp and Sowers [38] who examined the effects of highly specific antesera to gamma$_3$-MSH on the corticosterone response to ACTH in chronically cannulated rats. They showed that the alpha-$_3$-MSH antisera eliminated the ACTH induced rise of corticosterone. Human studies on the physiological significance of this peptide are lacking.

Growth Hormone

Colby et al [7] showed that growth hormone potentiated the effects of ACTH on adrenal function in hypophysectomized rats [7], but had no effect by itself on cortisol secretion. GH decreased 5 alpha reductase activity in the adrenal cortex. They suggested that the potentiating effect of GH on adrenocortical secretion occurred secondary to this effect [24]. Some of these effects may be related to alteration of hepatic metabolism of corticosterone by GH [6]. A physiological role for GH in regulating cortisol secretion in chronic stress has been suggested [1].

Serotonin

Krieger et al [25] had noted that cyproheptadine reduces hypercortisolemia in Cushing's Syndrome, probably due to its action on CNS serotonergic neurons. However, other studies have provided evidence that serotonin may have a direct effect on the the adrenal cortex [43]. Tait and Bradley [43] reported that serotonin at 8-10 uM increased corticosterone secretion in vitro. Raczk et al [32] reported that serotonin exerted a similar effect on isolated human adrenocortical cells. However, the physiological significance of serotonin in basal or stimulated cortisol secretion in humans, remains unclear.

Prostaglandins

Prostaglandins are present in the rat adrenal gland. Small doses of prostaglandins increased steroidogenesis in superfused adrenal glands obtained from hypophysectomized rats [14], an effect similar to that obtained with cyclic AMP [14]. Sarrita and Kaplan [36] reported that in many ways of prostaglandin stimulated corticosterone secretion similarly to ACTH; i.e., both responses are calcium-dependent, are inhibited by puromycin and both increased concentrations of cyclic AMP. Laychock et al suggest that the relationship between corticosterone production, ACTH and prostaglandins is complex and interlinked [27]. The physiological significance of prostaglandins in the HPA axis remains obscure.

Other ACTH potentiating substances

Factors derived from the thyroid, carcinomatous lung tissue and the liver have been shown to potentiate ACTH effects on steroidogenesis in isolated rat adrenal cells [29]. The exact character and nature of these factors has not been determined.

Immune-Adrenal Connection

Glucocorticoids have been known for many years to regulate various aspects of immune function. Recent studies suggest that two families of biologically active peptides of the type produced by immunogenic tissues influence adrenal steroidogenesis. One group is derived from the thymus gland. The ACTH-potentiating characteristic of thymosin fraction 5 was shown by several groups [20]. Thymosin factors induce maturation of T lymphocytes as their primary function. The other group of ACTH-potentiating factors belong to the class of lymphokines [3]. Again the exact nature of this factor remains controversial. It has been suggested that ACTH itself may be produced by the lymphocyte. The role and character of this lymphocyte-ACTH remains unknown. Blalock and Smith had also suggested that there was structural and functional homology between alpha-interferon and ACTH [3]. However, this has not been found by others. The role of alpha-interferon in regulating adrenocortical response is not known.

In summary, just as the regulatory mechanisms for ACTH release from the pituitary are increasingly recognized to be extremely complex, so also are the mechanisms regulating cortisol release from the adrenal. As a result, simplistic and direct inferences about the activity of the cephalic end of the HPA axis based on observed dysregulation of plasma cortisol in normals and depressed patients must be viewed with reservation.

ACKNOWLEDGMENTS

We are grateful to Elena Rowson for preparation of the manuscript. Supported by Clinical Associate Physician Award, NIH MH-RR0030, General Clinical Research Program, MH-42088, MH-40159 and MH-40524.

REFERENCES

1. Armanio A., Castellanos J. M., Balasch J. (1984): Horm. Metab. Res., 16 (3):142.

2. Axelrod J. (1962): J. Biol. Chem., 237:1657.

3. Blalock J. E., Smith E. M. (1980): Proc. Nat'l. Acad. Sci., 77:5972-5974.

4. Carroll B. J. (1982): Brit. J. Psychiatry, 40:292-304.

5. Carroll B. J., Curtis G. C., Mendels J. (1976): Arch. Gen. Psychiatry, 33:1039-1044.

6. Colby D., Gaskin J. H., Kitay J. I. (1974): Steroids, 24:679-686.

7. Colby D., Coffey J. L., Kitay J. I. (1973): Endocrinology, 93:188-192.

8. Endicott J., Spitzer R. L. (1979): American Journal of Psychiatry, 136:1,52-56.

9. Evans C. J., Erdelyi E., Weber E. and Barchas J. D. (1983): Science, 221:957.

10. Fehm H. L., Holl R., Klein E. and Voigt K. H. (1984): Klin Wochenschr, 62:19.

11. Fehm H. L. Holl R. Klein E., Voigt K. H. (1984): J. Clin. Endo. Metab., 58:410.

12. Fehm H. L., Holl R., Klein E., Voigt K. H. (1983): Clin. Physiol. Biochem., 1:329.

13. Feibel J. Kelly M. Lee L., Woolf P. (1983): J. Clin. Endocrinol. Metab., 57:1245.

14. Flack J. D., Jessup R., Ramwell P. W. (1969): Science, 163:691-692.

15. Garci-Alvarez F.M. (1979)L Anatomica (Zaragoza), 19:267.

16. Goeden M., Mantyh P. W., Hunt S. P., Emson P. C. (1984): Brain Research, 299:389.

17. Gold P. W., Chrousos G., Kellner C. et al (1984): Am. J. Psychiatry, 141:619-627.

18. Gullner H. G., Nicholson W. E., Wilson M. G., Bartter F. C., Orth D. N. (1982): Clin. Sc., 63:397.

19. Holsboer F., Doerr H. G., Sippell W. G. (1982): Acta.

Psychiat. Scand., 66:18-25.

20. Iida S., Itoh Y., Gomi M. Moriwaki K., Tarui S. (1984):
Hormone Res., 20.

21. Kiss T. (1951): Acta Anat. (Basel), 13:81.

22. Kolta M. G., Soliman K. F. A. (1981): Endokrinologie,
77:179.

23. Kolta M. G., Soliman K. F. A. (1981): Endocrin. Res.
Comm., 8 (4):239.

24. Kramer R. E., Greiner J. W., Colby H. D. (1977): Endocrinology, 101:297-303.

25. Krieger D. T. (1977): Ann. N. Y. Acad. Sci.,
297:527-534.

26. Krieger D. T., Allen W. (1975): J. Clin. Endo. Metab.,
10:675.

27. Laychock S. G., Warner W., Rubin R. P. (1977): Endocrinology, 100:74-81.

28. Lewis R. V., Stern A. S., Rossier J. (1979): Biochem.
Biophys. Research Communications, 89:822.

29. Matsuyama K., Moriwaki K., Iida S., Itoh Y., Gomi M.
Kawamura S., Tarui S. (1984): Endocrinol. Japan,
31:443.

30. Melchiorri P. (1980): In: Gastrointestinal Hormones,
edited by G. B. J. Glass, p. 717, Raven Press, New
York.

31. Pedersen, R. C., Browne A. C., Ling N. (1980):
Science, 208:1044.

32. Raczk K., Wolff I., Lada G. Y., Vida S., Glaz E.
(1979): Experientia, 35:1532-1533.

33. Ritchie J. C., Carroll B. C., Olton R. R., Shively V.,
Feinberg M. (1985): Archives of Gen. Psychiatry,
42:493-497.

34. Sachar E. J., Hellman L., Roffwarg H., Halpern F.,
Fukushima D., Gallagher T. (1978): Arch. Gen. Psychiatry, 28:19-24.

35. Sachar E. J., Hellman L, Fukushima D., Gallagher T.
(1973): Arch. Gen. Psychiatry 23:289-298.

36. Sarrita T., Kaplan N. M. (1972): Journal of Clinical
Investigation, 51:2246-2251.

37. Schteingart D. E., Conn J. W., Orth D. N., Harrison T. S., Fox J. E., Bookstein J. J. (1972): <u>J. Clin. Endo. Metab.</u>, 34:676.

38. Sharp B., Sowers J. R. (1983): <u>Biochem. and Biophy. Research Comm.</u>, 110:357.

39. Sherman, B. M., Schlecte J., Pfohl B. M. (1984): <u>Hormone Res.</u>, 20:157-165.

40. Soliman K. F. A. (1982): In: <u>Towards Chronopharmacology</u>, edited by R. Takaboshi, S. Halberg, and C. A. Walker, p 235. Pergamon Press, London.

41. Spitzer, R. L., Endicott, J. and Robins E. (1978): <u>Arch. of Gen. Psychiatry</u>, 35:773-782.

42. Suda T., Tomori N. Tozawa F., Demura H. Schizume K. Mouri T., Miura Y., Sasano N. (1984): <u>J. Clin. Endo. Metab.</u>, 58:919.

43. Taitt S. A., Bradley J. E. (1972): AJEB AK 50:833-887.

44. Unsicker K. (1951): <u>Z. Zellforsch</u>, 116:151.

45. Vogt M. (1947): <u>J. Physiol.</u>, 103:317.

46. Wetterberg L., Beck Friis J., Kjellmann B. F., Ljunggren J. G. (1984): In: <u>Frontiers in Biochemical and Pharmacological Research in Depression</u>, edited by E. Usdin, Raven Press, New York.

47. Wetzel R., Levine H. Hagman J., Ramachandran J. (1982): <u>Biochem. Biophys. Res. Commun.</u>, 104:944-947.

The Hypothalamic-Pituitary-Adrenal Axis: Physiology, Pathophysiology, and Psychiatric Implications, edited by A.F. Schatzberg and C.B. Nemeroff. Raven Press, Ltd., New York © 1988.

USE OF THE DEXAMETHASONE SUPPRESSION TEST IN CLINICAL PSYCHIATRY

Dwight L. Evans, M.D.

Department of Psychiatry
University of North Carolina School of Medicine
Chapel Hill, North Carolina 27514

INTRODUCTION

Considerable evidence now exists to suggest that dysregulation of the hypothalamic-pituitary-adrenal (HPA) axis occurs in patients with depression (14, 65). Earlier investigations found evidence of HPA hyperactivity in depression as manifested by elevated plasma cortisol (36, 49, 57, 58) and the dexamethasone suppression test (DST) was soon used as a more specific measure of the HPA axis (12, 13, 63, 64).

Much interest and controversy developed concerning the usefulness of the DST in clinical psychiatry following the publication by Carroll and associates (16) on the role of the DST as a specific biological marker for melancholia. Carroll and associates (16) reported a 67% sensitivity, 96% specificity, and 94% diagnostic confidence for the diagnosis of melancholia with the DST in psychiatric patients hospitalized on a research unit. Since this initial work (16) numerous studies have reported concordant (1, 2, 6, 18, 46, 47, 50, 59, 60) and discordant (4, 6, 22, 24, 55, 62, 66) findings.

Our group has studied the use of the DST in a non-research setting in order to determine the rate of DST non-suppression on a general adult and adolescent inpatient psychiatric unit using DSM-III diagnostic criteria in patients with depressive symptoms. We have also studied the use of the DST in patients hospitalized for an initial evaluation of cancer. The results of these clinical studies will be reported along with preliminary findings on the relationship between life events and the activity of the HPA axis as measured by the DST as well as preliminary findings regarding the effects of dexamethasone on immune status in major affective disorder.

CLINICAL FINDINGS

Major Depression

In order to determine the sensitivity and specificity for the diagnosis of major depression, the DST was administered to 166 consecutively admitted patients on our general inpatient, non-research psychiatric unit who either met DSM-III criteria for major affective disorder or had depressive symptoms associated with other DSM-III diagnoses. We studied 104 patients who met criteria for major depression (major depression without melancholia, n=62; major depression with melancholia, n=23; major depression with psychosis, n=19), seven diagnosed as schizoaffective, seven diagnosed as mixed

----

TABLE 1
RATES OF DEXAMETHASONE NON-SUPPRESSION IN PSYCHIATRIC INPATIENTS

| Diagnostic Group | N | % DST non-suppression | | | |
		>4	>5 (ug/dl)	>10	>15
"Depressive Symptoms" (A)	36	19	14	3	3
Major Depression - Total	104	72	63	38	14
- without melancholia (B)	62	60	48	21	6
- with melancholia (C)	23	87	78	43	9
- with psychosis (D)	19	95	95	84	47
Schizoaffective	7	43	43	29	0
Mania	6	33	33	33	33
Mixed Bipolar	7	100	100	43	14
Organic Affective Syndrome	6	67	67	33	33

Chi-squared analysis revealed the following significant differences between the diagnostic groups A, B, C, and D:
  B vs. A: $p < .001$ at 4 and 5 ug/dl, $p < .02$ at 10 ug/dl;
  C,D, vs. A: $p < .001$ at 4,5 and 10 ug/dl;
  D vs. A: $p < .001$ at 15 ug/dl;
  C vs. B: $p < .02$ at 4 and 5 ug/dl, $p < .04$ at 10 ug/dl;
  D vs. B: $p < .005$ at 4 ug/dl, $p < .001$ at 5, 10 and 15 ug/dl;
  C vs D: $p < .007$ at 10 ug/dl, $p < .004$ at 15 ug/dl.
(From The Journal of Psychiatric Research, in press. Reprinted by permission.)

----

bipolar disorder, six diagnosed as manic, six diagnosed as organic affective syndrome, and 36 who were classified as having "depressive symptoms", none of whom fulfilled criteria for major affective disorder (32). This study was a continuation of an earlier study which was reported in previous publications (25, 26, 27, 29).

The one mg DST was given and dexamethasone was administered at 11pm and blood samples were obtained the following day at 4pm and 11pm. Serum cortisol was assayed by specific radioimmunoassay procedures modified for sensitivity in the 2-8 ug/dl range. The medical exclusion criteria known to influence the DST (16) were used and non-suppression was defined as a post-dexamethasone serum cortisol > 5 ug/dl in either of the blood samples. (Other cutoff points were also evaluated.)

Sixty-six of the 104 patients with major depression (63%) showed dexamethasone non-suppression (>5 ug/dl criterion). Table 1 shows the rates of dexamethasone non-suppression in different diagnostic subgroups using different cutoff criteria as definitions of non-suppression. Five of 36 patients with "depressive symptoms" (14%) showed dexamethasone non-suppression and the DSM-III diagnoses in these 36 patients are listed in Table 2. A significantly higher percentage of patients with major depression showed

---

TABLE 2

DEXAMETHASONE SUPPRESSION TEST RESULTS IN PATIENTS WITH DEPRESSIVE SYMPTOMS AND DSM-III DIAGNOSES OTHER THAN MAJOR DEPRESSION

Diagnosis	N	Non-suppression	Percent
Adjustment Disorder with Depressed Mood	13	2	15
Schizophrenia	5	1	20
Dementia	3	1	33
Brief Reactive Psychosis	1	1	100
Post Traumatic Stress Disorder	3	0	0
Psychogenic Pain Disorder	3	0	0
Dysthymic Disorder	2	0	0
Somatoform Disorder	2	0	0
Schizotypal Personality	1	0	0
Schizophreniform Disorder	1	0	0
Organic Delusional	1	0	0
Generalized Anxiety Disorder	1	0	0
TOTAL	36	5	14

(From the Journal of Psychiatry Research, in press. Reprinted by permission.)

dexamethasone non-suppression than those patients with
"depressive symptoms". Among patients with major depression,
patients with major depression without melancholia showed
the lowest rate of DST non-suppression, whereas the patients
diagnosed as major depression with psychosis exhibited the
highest rate of DST non-suppression. The patients diagnosed
as major depression with melancholia showed a rate of DST
non-suppression greater than that seen in patients with
major depression without melancholia (4,5, and 10 ug/dl
cutoff) but less than that seen in the patients with
psychotic depression (10 and 15 ug/dl cutoff).

Figure 1 shows the mean serum cortisol concentrations
following dexamethasone in the different diagnostic sub
groups. The total major depression group had a higher mean
post dexamethasone serum cortisol level than the "depressive
symptoms" group and each of the subgroups of major
depression had higher mean serum cortisol concentrations
than the "depressive symptoms" group. The patients with
major depression with melancholia had higher mean cortisol
concentrations at 4pm than the patients with major
depression without melancholia and the patients with major
depression with psychosis had higher levels at 4 and 11pm
than the patients with major depression without melancholia,

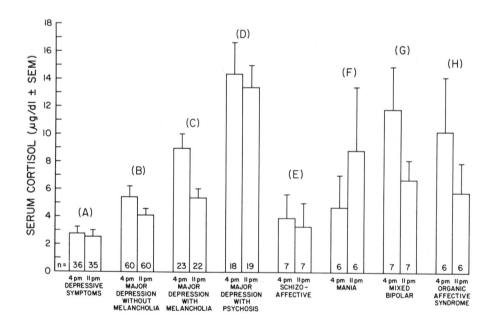

(From The Journal of Psychiatric Research, in press.
Reprinted by permission.)

as well as higher levels than the patients with major depression with melancholia. We found no significant relationship between post-dexamethasone serum cortisol values and patient's sex, nor any significant relationship between when the DST was done in relation to admission and serum cortisol values following dexamethasone.

We found the suggestion of a relationship between patient age and post dexamethasone cortisol levels, confirming a finding from our previous study (27). A small but significant relationship was found between post-dexamethasone cortisol levels (at 4pm but not 11pm) and patient age (Pearson r correlation +.17; p = 0.03) (Figure 2) However, no relationship existed when looking at the diagnostic sub groups separately. Further research will be necessary to assess the relationship between patient age and post-dexamethasone cortisol concentrations (10, 51, 68) and to assess any difference between age and post-dexamethasone cortisol levels between depressed patients and non-depressed controls (35, 42, 52).

These findings suggest a high incidence (63%) of dexamethasone non-suppression in patients with major depression. Moreover, significant differences in the rates of dexamethasone non-suppression as well as the post-

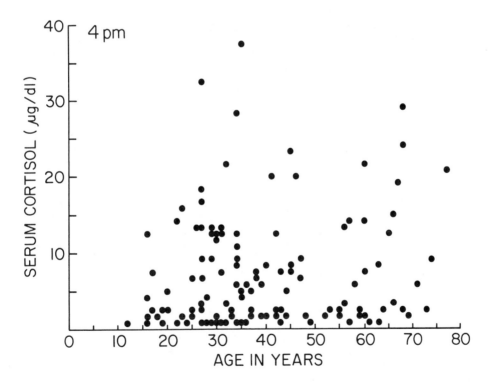

(From The Journal of Psychiatric Research, in press. Reprinted by permission.)

dexamethasone serum cortisol concentrations were found among the DSM-III sub groups of major depression. The patients with the most severe subtype of DSM-III major depression (melancholia) and particularly the patients with psychosis showed both the highest rate of dexamethasone non-suppression and the highest post-dexamethasone serum cortisol concentrations. If the 10 ug/dl criterion is used as a definition of non-suppression, 84% of the psychotic depressives could be identified compared to major depression with (43%) and without (21%) melancholia and compared to patients with depressive symptoms (3%). Furthermore, using a 15 ug/dl cutoff, 47% of the psychotic depressives showed non-suppression compared to major depression with (9%) and without (6%) melancholia and depressive symptoms (3%). These results are consistent with those of Schatzburg and associates (59) who found the highest rate of DST non-suppression as well as the highest post-dexamethasone serum cortisol concentrations in patients with psychotic depression. These findings could suggest that DST abnormality represents and increasing degree of severity of depression and/or a more biologically distinct subtype of depression.

It should be noted that although five of the 36 patients in the "depressive symptoms" group showed DST non-suppression, two patients with abnormal DST's went on to fulfill DSM-III criteria for major affective disorder and two other patients with abnormal DST's may have had a major affective disorder but were not diagnosed as such prior to the DST. The false positive DST rate would be 3% as opposed to the reported rate of 14% (32).

Organic Affective Syndrome

We found cortisol non-suppression after dexamethasone in four of six patients with organic affective syndrome and this is similar to the non-suppression rate observed in our major depressed patients (29, 30). Five of these patients fulfilled criteria for major depression and one was diagnosed schizoaffective (Table 3). Further study will be necessary to determine if the high frequency of cortisol non-suppression after dexamethasone in patients with a diagnosis of organic affective syndrome supports the concept that, regardless of the cause (endocrinopathy, altered neurochemical status, etc.), patients who fulfill criteria for major affective disorder may exhibit HPA axis hyperactivity.

Schizoaffective Disorder

Each of the seven patients with schizoaffective disorder exhibited both manic and depressive symptoms. Although three of the patients showed non-suppression of serum cortisol following dexamethasone, these three patients could not be differentiated on clinical grounds from the four schizoaffective disorder patients who showed normal

TABLE 3. CORTISOL RESPONSES TO DEXAMETHASONE IN PATIENTS WITH ORGANIC AFFECTIVE SYNDROME

Patient	Age (Years)	Sex	Organic Condition	Treatment	Clinical Response	Postdexamethasone Serum Cortisol Level (ug/dl)			
						Pre - Treatment 4pm	11pm	During Treatment 4pm	11pm
Nonsuppressors									
1	68	M	B12 Deficiency	B12	Excellent	23.9	13.2	2.1	2.7
2	77	F	B12 Deficiency hypothyroidism	B12; thyroxine haloperidol	Good	21.1	11.4	3.2	2.5
3	71	F	B12 Deficiency	B12; trazodone	Good	5.9	1.7	1.8[a]	
4	38	F	Hypothyroidism	Thyroxine chlorpromazine; lithium	Good	7.6	4.9		
Suppressors									
5	49	F	B12 deficiency hypothyroidism (euthyroid)	B12 thyroxine diphenylhydantoin; doxepin	Very good	1.0	1.8		
6	29	F	Hyperthyroidism	Methimazole Propylthiouracil; 131I; maprotiline; thiothixene	Good	1.1	1.2		

[a] Four months after discharge (predischarge 4 p.m. value, 5.7 ug/dl).

(From The American Journal of Psychiatry 141:1465–1467, 1984. Copyright 1984, the American Psychiatric Association. Reprinted by permission.)

suppression. It should be noted that five of the seven patients had been diagnosed previously as schizophrenic. Whether or not the DST identifies affective disorder in patients who are diagnosed schizophrenic requires further clinical research.

Bipolar Disorder

We have studied 13 patients with mania or mixed bipolar disorder. All seven of the patients with mixed bipolar disorder showed non-suppression of serum cortisol following dexamethasone (26). However, only two of six manic patients showed abnormal DST results. The two patients with an abnormal DST showed an irritable, dysphoric mood while the four patients with normal suppression showed an elevated, expansive, euphoric mood. We have suggested (28, 32), that dexamethasone non-suppression in bipolar disorder patients may be a characteristic of the mixed manic state as well as the irritable, dysphoric manic state but not the more classical euphoric manic state.

Dementia and Pseudodementia

We have preliminary findings in a small group of patients suggesting that the DST may identify major depression in patients with early and/or mild to moderate dementia. We have studied nine patients; pseudodementia (n=2); dementia (n=3); depression superimposed upon dementia (n=4). Both patients with major depression and mental status changes suggesting dementia exhibited cortisol non-suppression following dexamethasone and both patients exhibited normalization of the DST after successful antidepressant medication treatment; each patient showed complete resolution of both major depressive symptoms and the cognitive deficits (pseudodementia). Three of the four patients diagnosed as having both dementia and major depression showed cortisol non-suppression. All three of these patients showed cortisol suppression after successful antidepressant medication treatment. Each of the four patients underwent resolution of major depressive symptoms and three of the four patients experienced some improvement in cognitive functioning. One of the three patients diagnosed as having dementia and depressive symptoms (but not fulfilling DSM-III criteria for major depression) exhibited DST non-suppression. It should be noted that the DST findings in patients with dementia are variable (11, 21, 55, 62). Our finding of an abnormal DST in two patients with pseudodementia and normalization of the DST following successful antidepressant treatment taken together with the observation that the DST normalized after successful treatment of depression in all three of the dementia patients with concurrent major depression who exhibited DST non-suppression suggests that the DST may be useful in identifying major depression in patients with depressive pseudodementia as well as in patients with major depression superimposed upon dementia. However, we only studied three patients with dementia and without concurrent major depression and one of these patients showed an abnormal DST. The available studies (55, 62) suggest that the DST will be falsely positive in patients with advanced dementia and Grunhaus and colleagues (43) suggested that the severity and state of dementia may be better correlated with DST abnormality than dementia itself. Our findings are preliminary and additional study will be necessary to determine if the DST is useful in identifying major depression in patients with early and/or mild dementia.

The DST in Depressed Adolescents

We have administered the DST to 55 adolescents admitted to our inpatient psychiatric unit. Each of the adolescents showed significant depressive symptoms; 23 fulfilled DSM-III criteria for major depressive syndromes (20 major depression; 3 schizoaffective) and 32 fulfilled criteria for other DSM-III diagnoses (34). A significantly greater percentage of the adolescent patients with DSM-III major affective disorder showed serum cortisol non-suppression following dexamethasone than did those adolescent patients with other DSM-III diagnoses and depressive symptoms. (Table 4) Ten (43%) of the 23 patients with major depressive syndromes showed non-suppression. Five (16%) of the 32 patients with depressive symptoms showed an abnormal DST. We found no difference in the 4 and 11pm mean serum cortisol concentrations following dexamethasone between the major depressive syndrome group and the depressive symptoms group. It should be noted that of the five non-suppressors in the depressive symptom group, three eventually fulfilled criteria for major affective disorder and a fourth patient appeared to be a probable major depression. These follow up findings suggest that the DST identified major affective disorder in four of five adolescent patients who did not receive a major affective disorder diagnosis at the time of initial assessment. These findings are consistent with those of Targum and Capodanno (67) who suggested that the DST may be positive in adolescents who do not appear to meet DSM-III criteria for major depression but who later go on to manifest overt major affective disorders. In summary, we believe that the findings from this study in adolescents suggest that descriptive DSM-III criteria can be used to diagnose major depression in adolescent patients and furthermore that the DST may identify the presence of major depressive syndromes in some adolescent patients who have significant depressive symptoms but who do not appear on initial presentation to meet criteria for major depressive syndromes.

ANTIDEPRESSANT TREATMENT RESPONSE

Early investigations suggested that the DST may serve as a marker for a subtype of depression that responds well to biological treatment (8) and might predict the response to specific antidepressant medications (5, 7, 9, 41, 51). In a preliminary, open trial of 34 consecutively admitted patients with the DSM-III diagnosis of major depression treated with either maprotiline or trazodone, we found no significant difference in the antidepressant response rate between DST non-suppressors and suppressors. There was a trend for a greater response rate among non-suppressors (87% response rate) compared to suppressors (68% response rate). In addition, 6 of the 8 (75%) patients who did not respond to treatment showed dexamethasone suppression (61). We found no difference between maprotiline and trazodone on the response rate for suppressors or non-suppressors. Eighty-six percent of the non-suppressors responded to maprotiline and 88% of the non-suppressors responded to trazodone. Similarly, 70% of the suppressors responded to maprotiline and 67% of the suppressors responded to trazodone. In order to determine if this trend for a better response rate among DST non-suppressors is significant, and to determine if subtypes of major depression exist which are preferentially responsive to certain antidepressant medications, we are expanding the preliminary study to a larger number of patients who are being treated in a double blind fashion.

Table 4

DEXAMETHASONE SUPPRESSION TEST RESULTS
IN ADOLESCENT IN-PATIENTS

Diagnosis	N	Mean Age (years $\pm$ SD)	Age Range (years)	DST +[a] N	%
Major Affective Disorder[b]	23	15.3 $\pm$ 1.9	12-18	10	43
Depressive Symptoms	32	16.3 $\pm$ 2.1	12-19	5	16

[a] Non-suppression was defined as a serum cortisol level greater than 5 ug/dl at either 4 pm or 11 pm after 1 mg. dexamethasone the previous night.

[b] Significantly more of these patients exhibited non-suppression than did those patients with other diagnoses and depressive symptoms (p<.03, Fischer's Exact Probability Test).
(From Psychoneuroendocrinology, in press. Reprinted by permission.)

TREATMENT OUTCOME

Early data obtained from the DST indicated that non-suppression resolves with treatment (3, 8, 18, 40) and may predict the relative risk of relapse after treatment (38, 39, 40). In a study of 18 major depressed patients, we found that continued DST non-suppression was associated with poorer clinical response and increased risk of relapse compared to patients whose DST normalized (53). The 18 cortisol non-suppressors were retested before discharge and 13 patients demonstrated suppression at discharge while five patients did not. All of these suppressors exhibited a good to excellent response to drug treatment while four of the five non-suppressors showed only a fair to poor response to drug treatment. Only two of the 13 suppressors were readmitted compared to three of the five non-suppressors. In addition, one non-suppressor was transferred for continued inpatient treatment and the fifth non-suppressor became depressed four months after discharge. Thus, 80% of the patients who remained cortisol non-suppressors failed to improve or soon relapsed compared to 15% of the group of patients whose DST normalized. This relationship between normalization of the DST and a good to excellent clinical response was also observed in our patients with bipolar disorder, mixed type (26) and in patients with organic affective syndrome (29). Our results are consistent with the findings from two recent reviews (6, 20) which suggest that the DST could be a marker to monitor recovery from major depression. Further study will be necessary but this may be one of the most clinically relevant uses of the DST in clinical psychiatry (33).

DEPRESSION IN CANCER PATIENTS

In order to determine the prevalence of major depression in cancer patients and to assess the use of the DST and the thyrotropin releasing hormone (TRH) stimulation test for diagnosing depression in cancer patients, we studied 83 women hospitalized for gynecologic cancer (31). Nineteen (23%) were diagnosed to have a DSM-III major depression. The sensitivity and specificity of the DST (7 ug/dl criteria) for the diagnosis of major depression were 40% and 88%, respectively (Table 5). We found no relationship between DST and TRH results. Although the finding of a 40% sensitivity and 88% specificity of the DST for the diagnosis of DSM-III major depression suggests a potential clinical utility of the DST in identifying major depression in cancer patients, we excluded 28% of the patients screened because of the presence of medical factors known to influence the DST. This exclusion rate was approximately twice that found in our studies of psychiatric patients. These results suggest a high prevalence of depression in cancer patients but the relatively high exclusion rate for the DST could limit the potential clinical utility of the DST in cancer patients. Therefore, we believe the routine use of the DST in cancer patients to be premature at this time.

TABLE 5

RATES OF DST NONSUPPRESSION IN 47 HOSPITALIZED CANCER PATIENTS

		% DST Nonsuppression		
Diagnostic Group	N	With >5 ug/dl Criterion	With >7 ug/dl Criterion	With >10 ug/dl Criterion
Major Depression[a]	15	40	40	33
Nonmajor depression	11	27	18	9
Nondepressive disorder	3	67	0	0
No psychiatric diagnosis	18	17	11	6

[a] Fisher's exact test (one-tailed) revealed significant differences between the major depression group and the other three groups combined at 7 ug/dl (p<.05) and at 10 ug/dl (p<.03).
(From The American Journal of Psychiatry 143:447-452, 1986. Copyright 1986, the American Psychiatric Association. Reprinted by permission.)

MARGINAL HYPOTHYROIDISM AND THE DST

In an extension of our earlier study of antithyroid antibodies in depressed patients (54), we found a six fold increase (17% vs 3%) in the rate of of subclinical hypothyroidism (37) in depressed patients with DST non-suppression when compared to depressed patients with DST suppression (44). We also found a 17% rate of positive anti-thyroid antibody titers, confirming our earlier findings (54) and those of others (37, 56) which suggest that symptomless autoimmune thyroiditis may occur in a high percentage of patients hospitalized for affective disorders. We found no relationship between the presence of antithyroid antibodies and DST status. The high rate of subclinical hypothyroidism in patients with affective syndromes suggest that patients with affective disorders may benefit from a complete thyroid evaluation and that affective disorder patients who show DST non-suppression may benefit particularly from this thyroid evaluation. We are now extending this study to include TRH testing which will permit a more refined thyroid assessment to assess the potential association between the HPT axis and the HPA axis as assessed by the DST.

PRELIMINARY FINDINGS

Life Experience, Major Affective Disorder, and the DST

We observed anecdotally a strong relationship between DST non-suppression and a history of object loss in patients who presented with symptoms of mixed bipolar disorder. We have preliminary findings from a retrospective review of 96 patients with major affective disorder. We found a preponderance of early loss (death of a parent before age 20) in patients with mixed mania when compared to patients with dysphoric mania and euphoric mania, though dexamethasone non-suppression appeared to be related to diagnosis rather than to a history of loss (Table 6). Although there was a similar incidence of loss when comparing patients with major depression to patients with depressive symptoms, the melancholic subtype of major depression appears to be associated with an increased incidence of both early and later loss when compared to

TABLE 6
LOSS, DST AND MANIA

	N	Loss (%) Early	Later	Total	+DST (%)
Mixed Mania	14	21	43	64	71
Dysphoric Mania	13	0	38	38	61
Mania	5	0	40	40	20

TABLE 7
LOSS, DST AND MAJOR AFFECTIVE DISORDER

	N	LOSS(%) EARLY	LATER	TOTAL	+DST (%)
Depressive Symptoms	12	17	33	50	8
Major Depression	49	14	21	35	57
- Melancholia	35	9	20	29	43
+ Melancholia	10	30	30	60	90
+ Psychosis	4	25	0	25	100
Mania	35	11	40	51	63

depressed patients without melancholia. Once again there
appears to be no consistent relationship between loss
history and DST status (Table 7).

We also have preliminary findings on the relationship
between early and recent abuse (physical and sexual) and HPA
activity as measured by the DST. Cole (23) studied the
prevalence and extent of abuse in patients admitted to our
psychiatry service here at the University of North Carolina
Memorial Hospital. Preliminary analyses of a collaborative
study done with Cole suggest that there is a lower rate of
DST non-suppression in female major affective disorder
patients who have suffered both child and adult abuse
compared to female patients who suffered no abuse or who
suffered abuse either in childhood or adulthood alone (Table
8). Our findings suggest also that the post dexamethasone
serum cortisol levels were significantly lower in major
affective disorder female patients who had extrafamilial
sexual abuse whereas the post-dexamethasone serum cortisol
levels were significantly elevated in major affective
disorder patients who had experienced marital rape.

TABLE 8
ABUSE, DST AND MAJOR AFFECTIVE DISORDER

	No Abuse +DST	Child + Adult Abuse +DST	Child Abuse +DST	Adult Abuse +DST
Major Depression	58%(7/12)	20%(2/10)*	100%(3/3)	100% (1/1)
Major Affective Disorder	58% (7/12)	17% (2/12)**	100%(3/3)	100% (1/1)
Other Disorders	------	0% (0/4)	25%(1/4)	0% (0/1)
All Diagnoses	58% (7/12)	13 (2/16)***	57%(4/7)	50% (1/2)

```
 * = p < .10        Child + Adult Abuse
** = p < .05               vs.
*** = p < .02           No Abuse
```

Sensitivity of the Immune System to Corticosteroids in Depression

Although depression is associated with HPA hyperactivity
and hypercortisolism, depressed patients with elevated post-
dexamethasone serum cortisol levels do not show the physical

TABLE 9

DEXAMETHASONE EFFECTS: ADMISSION VS DISCHARGE

THE MAGNITUDE OF CHANGE IN NUMBERS (x 10^3) OF WBCS,
TOTAL LYMPHOCYTES AND SUBPOPULATIONS OF T LYMPHOCYTES
AFTER DEXAMETHASONE ADMINISTRATION (1 MG) IN INPATIENTS
WITH MAJOR AFFECTIVE DISORDER WHEN ILL (AT ADMISSION)
OR AFTER RECOVERY (AT DISCHARGE)

	MAJOR AFFECTIVE DISORDER	
	ADMISSION (n=16)	DISCHARGE (n=6)
ER's	$0.04 \pm .14$	$-0.43 \pm .19*$ p < .08
LEU2	$0.05 \pm .04$	$-0.05 \pm .04$
LEU3	$0.00 \pm .08$	$-0.30 \pm .09**$ p < .02
LEU4	$-0.02 \pm .14$	$-0.41 \pm .14**$ p < .03
LEU7	$0.02 \pm .01$	$-0.02 \pm .02$
LEU 11	$0.04 \pm .02**$ p < .03	$-0.02 \pm .02$
SIG	$0.00 \pm .03$	$-0.07 \pm .06$
WBC	$1.66 \pm .33**$ p < .001	$1.30 \pm .27**$ p < .01
Lymph	$-0.02 \pm .17$	$-0.49 \pm .22*$ p< .08

* = trend change, ** significant change
(comparison postdexamethasone vs predexamethasone immune
values; paired t-tests)

The total number $\pm$SEM (x10^3) of white blood cells
(WBC), lymphocytes and lymphocyte subpopulations
identified by E- rosetting (ERs) and· by tagging with
monoclonal antibodies against various T lymphocyte
surface proteins (Leu 2, Leu 3, Leu 4, Leu 7, Leu 11
obtained from Becton-Dickinson) shortly after admission
to hospital in patients with major depression, major
affective disorder (major depression and bipolar
disorder) or non-major affective disorders. Measurement
of percent of lymphocytes tagged by each antibody was
done using flow cytometry. E-rosettes and Leu 4 are
approximate measures of the total number of T
lymphocytes. Leu 2 is an approximate measure of the
population of suppressor T cells. Leu 3 is an
approximate measure of the population of helper T
cells. Leu 7 and 11 are approximate measures of natural
killer cell populations.

----

stigmata of Cushings Syndrome. Lowy et al (48) suggested that the chronic elevations of serum cortisol in depression might be associated with a reduction in glucocorticoid receptor sensitivity or function throughout the body. These authors found that a 1 mg dose of dexamethasone administered as part of the DST was associated with decreased T-cell mitogen stimulation. This reduction in lymphoproliferative response was seen in control subjects and depressed patients who showed normal suppression to dexamethasone. However, dexamethasone had no effect on the T-cell mitogen stimulation response in patients who showed non-suppression of serum cortisol by dexamethasone. In addition, the degree of immune suppression as measured by mitogen stimulation was negatively correlated with the post-dexamethasone serum cortisol levels. Although there was no relationship between the pre-dexamethasone serum cortisol levels and the post-dexamethasone mitogen stimulation results, Lowy et al (48) suggested that the lymphocyte resistance to dexamethasone could result from a down regulation of the glucocorticoid receptors in response to elevated serum levels of cortisol.

We have studied the effects of dexamethasone on T-cell numbers and T-cell subset numbers and found significant differences after admission compared to discharge DSTs (Table 9). Major affective disorder patients had a significant increase in the number of natural killer cells following one mg of dexamethasone on admission (n=16) but had significant decreases in total T-cell numbers and T-helper cell numbers following dexamethasone prior to discharge when clinically well (n=6) (31). These findings suggest a state related immune resistance to corticosteroids in patients with major affective disorder.

We are now extending this work by studying the sensitivity of lymphocytes to glucocorticoids by assessing the effects of dexamethasone on T-cell and T-cell subset numbers as well as T-cell activity, including mitogen stimulation, mitogen stimulated lymphokine production, and natural killer cell activity. We are also measuring 24 hour urinary free cortisol to assess more completely the relationship between hypercortisolism and lymphocyte sensitivity to glucocorticoids. We are studying patients after recovery from major depression in order to assess the state dependent nature of the cortisol-immune relationship.

CONCLUSIONS

The DST has received extensive research study and has been used in clinical psychiatry as a potential marker of major depression. Although the sensitivity of the DST for the diagnosis of depression has varied among the available studies, the DST appears to be moderately sensitive for the diagnosis of major affective disorder and approximately 50% of major affective disorder patients will have an abnormal DST. Our findings taken from the clinical inpatient setting, suggest that the rate of DST abnormality increases across the range of patients going from patients with depressive symptoms (14%) to major depression without melancholia (48%), to major depression with melancholia (78%), and through major depression with psychosis (95%) (32). These findings are confirmed by the results of a recent review of over 5000 patients (6) where the rate of DST non-suppression increased across the range of normal controls, acute grief, dysthymic disorders, through major depression without melancholia, major depression with melancholia, major depression with psychosis, mixed mania, and severely suicidal depressives. In addition, we have found not only an increasing rate of DST non-suppression, but also a higher absolute post-dexamethasone serum cortisol concentration across the range from depressive symptoms, major depression without melancholia, major depression with melancholia, and major depression with psychosis. Further research will be necessary to determine if DST non-suppression represents an increasing degree of severity of affective disorder and/or a more biologically distinct subtype of affective disorder.

The DST may have a particular use as a marker of treatment response in depressed patients who have an abnormal DST during the depressed state. Our results suggest that continued non-suppression (failure to normalize) may be associated with poor clinical outcome and increased risk of relapse. Further longitudinal study will be necessary to determine if the DST can be used as a marker of relapse in patients who develop an abnormal DST after having normalized the DST upon recovery previously.

Our findings suggest that the DST may be useful in identifying major affective disorder in patients who do not meet full DSM-III criteria for major affective disorder at the time of the initial admission, but who go on to develop overt evidence of affective disorder. In addition, the DST may be useful in identifying those adolescent patients who show atypical signs and symptoms of affective disorder and who later meet descriptive criteria for affective disorder. If further research confirms these findings, earlier recognition and treatment of affective disorder might be possible in patients with atypical affective presentations and abnormal DST results.

A biological marker for depression would be particularly useful in the clinical assessment of depression in non-psychiatric patients. For example, the signs and symptoms of major depression are often difficult to diagnose in patients with cancer. We found a high prevalence of depression in patients with cancer and also found a 40% sensitivity and an 88% specificity of the DST for major depression in this population. However, the medical exclusion rate was sufficiently high to suggest that the DST should not be used routinely in the assessment of depression in cancer patients.

Our findings suggest also that the DST may be useful in assessing the activity of the HPA axis and the relationship of this endocrine axis to the HPT axis. Depressed patients with DST non-suppression were found to have a higher rate of marginal hypothyroidism. Thus, affective disorder patients with DST non-suppression may benefit particularly from evaluation of thyroid status.

We also have pilot data which suggest no relationship between a history of early or recent loss and hyperactivity of the HPA axis as measured by the DST. However, further study is necessary to measure a broader range of losses and life events as well as the assessment of personality function and the social support systems that prevail at the time of loss. Loss may have different biological and psycho logical consequences depending on the type of loss, timing of the loss, the family-social system, and the personality of the individual. Our preliminary findings suggest a relationship between the activity of the HPA axis and physical and sexual abuse. Further study also will be necessary to assess the relationship between the HPA axis and physical and/or sexual abuse as well as the relationship with loss and other traumatic life events.

Our preliminary findings on the effects of dexamethasone on the immune system in patients with major affective disorder suggest a state related immune resistance to glucocorticoids in major affective disorder. The DST could prove useful in further studies assessing the endocrine and immune relationships in major affective disorder.

Finally, the work presented here forms the foundation for the long term objective of assessing the inter-relationships between the endocrine and immune systems in major affective disorders and in physical illnesses. A better understanding of the immune changes in major affective disorder and the relationship with the HPA axis as well as other endocrines should indicate if these immune and endocrine changes are clinically relevant and if they play a role in the development of physical diseases. Because alterations in immune function (as related to endocrine function and as related to life experience and psychological pstate) could effect the development and course of physical illness (such as cancer), we plan to assess in future studies the relationship between psychological state, neuroendocrine-immune state, and the course of cancer in patients with malignancies. The DST, as a measure of HPA axis activity and as a challenge to the immune system, should prove useful in these future investigations.

ACKNOWLEDGEMENTS

This work was supported in part by National Institute of Mental Health - Mental Health and Clinical Research Center Grant MH33127.

REFERENCES

1. Aggernaes, H., Kirkegaard, C., Krog-Meyer, I., Kijne, B., Larsen, J.K., Lund Laursen, A., Lykke-Olesen, L., Mikkelsen, P.L., Rasmussen, S., and Bjorum, N. (1983): Acta Psychiatr Scand 67:258-264.

2. Agren, H. and Wide, L. (1982): Psychoneuroendocrinol. 7:309-327.
3. Albala, A.A., Greden, J.F., Tarika, J., and Carroll, B.J. (1981): Biol. Psychiatry 16:551-560.
4. Amsterdam, J.D., Winokur, A., Caroff, S.N., and Conn, J. (1982): Am J Psychiatry 139:3:287-291.
5. Amsterdam, J.D., Winokur, A., Lucki, I., Caroff, S., Snyder, P., and Rickels, K. (1983): Arch Gen Psychiatry 40:515-521.
6. Arana, G.W., Baldessarini, R.J., and Ornsteen, M. (1985): Arch Gen Psychiatry 42:1193-1204.
7. Beckmann, H., Holzmuller, B., and Fleckenstein, P. (1984): Acta Psychiatr Scand 70:341-353.
8. Brown, W.A. and Shuey, I. (1980): Arch Gen Psychiatry 37:747-751.
9. Brown, W.A., Haier, R.J., Qualls, C.B. (1980): Lancet 1: 928-929.
10. Brown W.A. (1982): Am J Psychiatry 139:1376-1377.
11. Carnes, M., Smith, J.C., Kalin, N.H., and Bauwens, S.F. (1983): Psychiatry Research 9:337-344.
12. Carroll, B.J., Martin, F.I.R., Davies, B.M. (1968): Br Med J 3:285-287.
13. Carroll, B.J., and Davies, B.M. (1970): Br Med J 1:789-791.
14. Carroll, B.J. and Mendels, J. (1976): In: Hormones, Behavior and Psychopathology. Edited by E.J. Sachar, New York, Raven Press.
15. Carroll, B.J., Greden, J.F., Feinberg, M., Lohr, N., James, N., Steiner, M., Haskett, R.F., Albala, A.A., DeVigne, J.P., and Tarika, J. (1981): Psychiatric Clinics of North America 4:89-99.
16. Carroll, B.J., Feinberg, M., Greden, J.F., Tarika, J., Albala, A.A., Haskett, R .F., James, N.M., Kronfol, Z., Lohr, N., Steiner, M., de Vigne, J.P., and Young, E. (1981): Arch Gen Psychiatry 38:15-22.
17. Carroll, B.J., Greden, J.F., and Feinberg, M. (1981): In: Recent Advances in Neuropsychopharmacology. Edited by B. Angrist, Pergamon Press, Oxford.
18. Carroll, B.J. (1982): Brit J Psychiatry 140:292-304.
19. Carroll, B.J. (1983): J Clin Psychiatry 44:30-40.
20. Carroll, B.J. (1985): J Clin Psychiatry 46:13-24.
21. Castro, P., Lemaire, M., Toscano-Aguilar, M., and Herchuelz, A. (1983): Am J Psychiatry 140:386.
22. Ceulemans, D.L., Westenberg, H.G., and van Pragg, H.M. (1985): Psychiatry Research 14:189-195.
23. Cole, C. (In Press): The Clinical Social Work Journal.
24. Dewan, M.J., Pandurangi, A.K., Boucher, M.L., Levy, B.F., and Major, L.F. (1982): Am J Psychiatry 139:1501-1503.
25. Evans, D.L. and Nemeroff, C.B. (1983a): Biological Psychiatry 18: 505-511.
26. Evans, D.L. and Nemeroff, C.B. (1983b): Am J Psychiatry 140:615-617.
27. Evans, D.L., Burnett, G.B., and Nemeroff, C.B. (1983): Am J Psychiatry 140:586-589.

28. Evans, D.L. and Nemeroff, C.B. (1984a): Am J Psychiatry 141:146-147.
29. Evans, D.L. and Nemeroff, C.B. (1984b): Am J Psychiatry 141:1465-1467.
30. Evans, D.L. and Nemeroff, C.B. (1985): Am J Psychiatry 142:992.
31. Evans, D.L., McCartney, C.F., Nemeroff, C.B., Raft, D., Quade, D., Golden, R.N., Haggerty, J.J., Holmes, V., Simon, J.S., Droba, M., Mason, G.A., and Fowler, W.C. (1986): Am J Psychiatry 143:447-452.
32. Evans, D.L. and Nemeroff, C.B. (in press): J Psych Research.
33. Evans, D.L. and Golden, R.N. (in press): In: Handbook of Clinical Psychoneuroendocrinology, edited by C.B. Nemeroff and P.T. Loosen, Guilford Press, New York.
34. Evans, D.L., Nemeroff, C.B., Haggerty, J.J., and Pedersen, C.A. (in press): Psychoneuroendocrinology.
35. Fogel, B.S., and Satel, S.L. (1985): J Clin Psychiatry 46:95-97.
36. Gibbons, J.L., and McHugh, P.R. (1963): J Psychiatry Res 1:162-171.
37. Gold, M.S., Pottash, A.L.C., and Extein, I. (1982): Psychiatry Research 6:261-269.
38. Goldberg, I.K. (1980): Lancet 1:376.
39. Goldberg, I.K. (1980b): Lancet 2:92.
40. Greden, J.F., Albala, A.A., Haskett, R.F., James, N.M., Goodman, L., Steiner, M., and Carroll, B.J. (1980): Biological Psychiatry 15:449-458.
41. Greden, J.F., Kronfol, Z., Gardner, R., Feinberg, M., Mukhopadhyay, S., Albala, A., and Carroll, B. (1981): J Affect Dis 3:389-396.
42. Greden, J.F., Tiongco, D., Haskett, R.F., Grunhaus, L., and Kotun, J. (1986): Presented at 41st Annual Meeting Society of Biological Psychiatry, Washington, D.C., No. 155.
43. Grunhaus, L., Dilsaver, S., Greden, J.F., and Carroll, B.J. (1983): Biological Psychiatry 18:215-225.
44. Haggerty, J.J., Simon, J.S., Nemeroff, C.B., and Evans, D.L.. (1986): Presented at 41st Annual Meeting, Society of Biological Psychiatry Annual Meeting, Washington, D.C. No. 181.
45. Hallstrom, T., Samuelsson, S., Ballsin, J., Walinder, J., Bengtsson, C., Nystrom, E., Andersch, B., Lindstedt, G., and Lundberg, P. (1983): Br J Psychiatry 142:489-497.
46. Holden, N.L. (1983): Br J Psychiatry 142:505-512.
47. Kasper, S. and Beckmann, H. (1983): Acta Psychiat Scan 68:31-37.
48. Lowy, M.T., Reder, A.T., Antel, J.P., and Meltzer, H.Y. (1984): Am. J. Psychiatry 141:1365-1370.
49. McClure, D.J. (1966): J Psychosom Res 10:189- 195.
50. Mendlewicz, J., Charles, G., and Frankson, J.M. (1982): Br J Psychiatry 141:464-470.
51. Nelson, W.H., Orr, W.W., Stevenson, J.M., and Shane, S.R. (1982); Arch Gen Psychiatry 39:1033-1036.

52. Nelson, W.H., Khan, A., Orr, W.W., and Tanragouri, R.N. (1984): Biological Psychiatry 19: 1293-1304.
53. Nemeroff, C.B., and Evans, D.L. (1984): Am. J. Psychiatry 141:247-249.
54. Nemeroff, C.B., Simon, J.S., Haggerty, J.J., and Evans, D.L. (1985): Am. J. Psychiatry 142:840-843.
55. Raskind, M., Peskind, E., Rivard, M.F., Veith, R., and Barnes, R. (1982): Am J Psychiatry 139:1468-1471.
56. Reus, V.I., Berlant, J., Galante, M., and Becker, N. (1986): Presented at 41st Annual Meeting, Society of Biological Psychiatry, Washington, D.C., No. 39.
57. Sachar, E.J. (1967a): Arch Gen Psychiatry 17:544-553.
58. Sachar, E.J. (1967b): Arch Gen Psychiatry 17:554-557.
59. Schatzberg, A.F., Rothchild, A.J., Stahl, J.B., Bond, T.C., Rosenbaum, A.H., Lofgren, S.B., McLaughlin, R.A., Sullivan, M.A., and Cole, J.O. (1983): Am J Psychiatry 140:88-91.
60. Schlesser, M.A., Winokur, G., and Sherman, B.M. (1980): Arch Gen Psychiatry 37:737-743.
61. Simon, J.S., Nemeroff, C.B., and Evans, D.L. (1986): Presented at 41st Annual Meeting of the Society of Biological Psychiatry, Washington, D.C., No. 191.
62. Spar, J.E. and Gerner, R. (1982): Am J Psychiatry 139:238-240
63. Stokes, P.E. (1966): The Endocrine Society (USA), 48th Meeting Abstracts, Endocrinology 78: (suppl.).
64. Stokes, P.E. (1972): In : Recent Advances in the Psychobiology of the Depressive Illnesses. Edited by T.A. Williams, M.M. Katz, and J.A. Shield, Washington, DC: US Government Printing Office.
65. Stokes, P.E., Pick, G.R., Stoll, P.M., and Nunn, W.D. (1975): J Psychiatry Res 12:271-281.
66. Stokes, P.E., Stoll, P.M., Koslow, S.H., Maas, J.W., Davis, J.M., Swann, A.C., and Robins, E. (1984): Arch Gen Psychiatry 41:257-267.
67. Targum, S.D. and Capodanno, A.E. (1983): Am J Psychiatry 140:589-591.
68. Tourigny-Rivard, M.F., Raskind, M., and Rivard, D. (1981): Biological Psychiatry 16:1177-1184.

The Hypothalamic-Pituitary-Adrenal Axis:
Physiology, Pathophysiology, and Psychiatric
Implications, edited by A.F. Schatzberg and
C.B. Nemeroff. Raven Press, Ltd., New York
© 1988.

WHY DEXAMETHASONE RESISTANCE? TWO POSSIBLE NEUROENDOCRINE MECHANISMS

Robert M. Sapolsky
Department of Biological Sciences
Stanford University
Stanford, CA 94305

and

Bruce S. McEwen
Laboratory of Neuroendocrinology
Rockefeller University
1230 York Avenue
New York, NY 10021

The demonstration of dexamethasone (DEX) resistance in certain depressive patients was a particularly exciting finding for biological psychiatry. The endocrine abnormality strengthened the perception of biological underpinnings in affective disorders; such a perception is, of course, a raison d'etre of biological psychiatry. Furthermore, that only some patients were DEX resistant gave endocrine credence to the longstanding view of the heterogeneity of affective disorders, and promised to provide a new diagnostic tool for meaningfully sub-typing depressive individuals.

With time, however, some of this enthusiasm has waned. While there have been some reports that outcome of the DST can be predictive of the course and outcome of the disorder (9,41), this has often been disappointing (15,18,42). In addition, the correlations between DEX resistance and depressive sub-types have not been strong enough to provide the clear-cut diagnostic tool that some envisioned earlier. Finally, while the endocrine abnormality of DEX resistance still testifies to the biological reality of affective disorders, it is not yet clear what exactly that reality is.

In this chapter, we will consider this final issue. On a very mechanistic neuroendocrine level, what changes in the adrenocortical axis underlie DEX resistance? We will review the physiological and demographic features of DEX resistance in the depressive and in the sufferer of Alzheimer's Disease (AD). We do so only briefly, given its treatment throughout this volume, as well as the presumed familiarity of most readers with its features. We will then review an experimental rodent and primate literature which suggests two different routes by which DEX resistance and, more generally, hypercortisolism can arise. The first model, we will argue, may be analogous to the situation in AD, while the second might explain the transient DEX resistance of some depressives. Specifically, we propose that:

1. The hippocampus is one of the suprahypothalamic sites in the limbic system which inhibits the adrenocortical axis. Such inhibition represents, at least in part, negative feedback by circulating glucocorticoids (GCs) upon the axis. Glucocorticoids exert their inhibitory effects via interactions with corticosteroid receptors in hippocampal neurons.

2.   Destruction of the hippocampus, or of its efferents, produces a syndrome of hypercortisolism, because of disruption of GC negative feedback. Such a syndrome can include elevated basal or post-stress GC secretion, disrupted circadian rhythmicity of the axis, and resistance to feedback suppression. The features of hypercortisolism in the AD patient may arise from the hippocampal degeneration typical of the disorder.

3.   A depletion of corticosteroid receptors in the hippocampus (with no damage done to the neurons themselves) desensitizes the hippo-campus to a GC negative feedback signal and thus also produces a syndrome of hypercortisolism. Such receptors can be depleted by pro-longed stress, as stress-induced elevations in circulating GC concen-trations down-regulate the number of corticosteroid receptors. The hippocampus' complement of these receptors appears to be the most vulnerable in the brain to such stress-induced down-regulation. With the abatement of stress, receptor concentrations (and hippocampal neuroendocrine function) normalizes. The features of hypercortisolism in some depressive patients may reflect transient down-regulation of the concentrations of such receptors.

Hypercortisolism in the depressive and AD patient

The first report of hypercortisolism in the depressive came in 1963 (38). Since then, an array of hypercortisolemic features have been demonstrated to occur in approximately 50% of individuals. Basal con-centrations of cortisol can be elevated quite dramatically in some cases, even to within the range seen with Cushing's syndrome (14,15,68,77,78). Sachar and colleagues (79) demonstrated that this hypersecretion is most pronounced from late afternoon to evening, during what should normally be the circadian trough in cortisol secre-tion. Along with the basal hypersecretion came reports of impaired sensitivity of the axis to feedback inhibition, namely the continued secretion of cortisol despite what should be a strong inhibitory signal induced by DEX (10,14,90,97). Most strictly defined (15), DEX resist-ance is considered to occur when a 1 mg dose of DEX fails to suppress cortisol concentrations to less than 5 $\mu g/dl$ 17 and 24 hours later. Others have found additional, more subtle forms of impaired feedback sensitivity, in that the criteria of suppressed cortisol concentrations may be achieved, but either more slowly or more transiently (i.e., "early escape" from suppression) (92). It has become clear that depressive hypercortisolism, as expressed by elevated basal cortisol concentrations, and as expressed by DEX resistance, need not always occur together in the same individual (3,44,97). We will return to this point at the end of the chapter.

The anatomical locus of the hypersecretion is only recently becom-ing understood. Potentially, the phenomenon could be entirely peripheral; i.e., adrenal hypersecretion of cortisol in response to a normal ACTH signal. However, the demonstration that depressive hyper-cortisolism is often accompanied by hypersecretion of ACTH (51,74) moves the onus of abnormality to the level of the pituitary or brain (although it should be noted that ACTH hypersecretion is not always observed [29]). If, as we shall argue, the defect is substantially within the CNS, concentrations of corticotropin releasing factor (CRF) (and/or the other secretagogues that facilitate ACTH release, including vasopressin [VP], oxytocin and catecholamines) should be elevated within the hypothalamic portal blood of hypercortisolemic depressives. Obviously, this is not possible to determine.   However, it has been demonstrated recently that CRF concentrations are elevated in the CSF of depressives (68).   While portal concentrations of the peptide cannot be accurately inferred from CSF concentrations, this finding indirectly supports the   notion of primary CNS hypersecretion under-lying depressive hypercortisolism.   Two additional studies (39,46) support this conclusion.   Both reported that the pituitary response to CRF is blunted in depressives. Furthermore the extent of such blunting tended to be positively correlated with the severity of hypercortisol-ism. The attenuated response to CRF could occur because the elevated cortisol concentrations exert an exaggerated inhibitory feedback effect upon the pituitary.   Thus, failure of feedback regulation at the pituitary level cannot be occurring, and the onus of insensitivity and hypersecretion is shifted to the CNS. Alternatively or additionally, the attenuated response to CRF could occur because of chronic hyper-secretion of CRF, with the pituitary becoming less sensitive to the peptide as an only partially successful compensation. Again, the onus of hypersecretion falls upon the CNS.   These studies, while indirect, support the idea that depressive hypercortisolism arises from a primary CNS defect.

As noted, the original optimism of some in expecting that the DST would be a means to conclusively differentiate between depressive sub-types has not been borne out.   However, certain patterns have emerged. A higher incidence of nonsuppression has been identified in familial pure depressive disease, as compared with either sporadic depression or depression spectrum disease (105).   Moreover, psychotic depression is also associated with a high rate of DEX resistance (27,28,79,89). Finally, a particularly convincing correlate of hypercortisolism in depression appears to be senescence.   A recent spate of papers have shown that in both genders and in a number of different depressive subtypes, DEX resistance and/or hypercortisolism becomes more prevalent in older populations (3,34,36,44,60,69,77,97).   One such report showed fully 83% of aged (over 60 years of age) depressives were DEX resistant (36). We shall return to the significance of this age factor below.

A similar syndrome of hypercortisolism occurs in AD. This includes both hypersecretion of cortisol under basal conditions, as well as DEX resistance (4,12,13,73,96). Approximately 50% of AD patients show some form of hypercortisolism.   Interestingly, as with depression, the incidence of hypercortisolism increases with age among AD patients (43).

The hippocampus as an inhibitor of the HPA axis

Corticotropin releasing factor is released by the hypothalamus in small amounts during non-stressed times under the control of circadian CNS oscillators, and in larger quantities in response to stress. Circulating through the hypothalamic-hypophysial portal system, CRF stimulates the release of ACTH from pituitary corticotrophs.   In addition, other secretagogues such as VP, oxytocin and catecholamines are secreted during stress, have some ability to directly release ACTH and, more significantly, synergize with CRF in releasing ACTH. ACTH, in turn, releases GCs from the adrenal cortex (75).

Feedback inhibition is a critical component of the regulation of this cascade. The principal inhibitory influence comes from GCs, in that they inhibit subsequent secretion at every step in the system. Thus, this constitutes a classical case of end-product inhibition.

Such GC feedback inhibition is vastly complex. Within a short time period (less than an hour), it is the rate of change of circulating GC concentration that determines the extent of inhibition of subsequent secretion (rate sensitive fast feedback). Over longer time domains, it is the absolute level of GC concentrations achieved which is most predictive of inhibition (level sensitive delayed feedback). Over the shorter time domain, inhibition primarily involves depressed secretion of pre-existing stores of relevant hormones; over the longer time periods of feedback, inhibition of hormone synthesis becomes involved also. The strength and precise temporal parameters of these different forms of GC feedback vary, depending on whether one considers GC-induced inhibition of basal adrenocortical activity, or of stress-induced activity. The reader is directed to Keller-Wood and Dallman (55) for a comprehensive review of this difficult subject.

The anatomical loci of such feedback is our primary concern in this section. Glucocorticoid-feedback inhibition can occur at the pituitary level. This can be shown in hypothalamic-lesioned animals in whom pituitary responsiveness to CRF is diminished by a GC feedback signal (49). Similar feedback can be demonstrated at the purely hypothalamic level, utilizing hypothalamic explants (25,45).

Combining these components, it is clear that a bulk of GC feedback occurs at the levels of the hypothalamus and pituitary (55). However, this is not all, and suprahypothalamic sites within the CNS also mediate some of the feedback signal. This can be shown most directly by surgically de-afferenting the medial basal hypothalamus (i.e., forming a hypothalamic "island"). The efficacy of synthetic GCs in suppressing adrenocortical activity is reduced--in effect, such rats are relatively DEX resistant (30).

Of potential suprahypothalamic inhibitory sites, the hippocampus has been most frequently implicated. While such evidence has been accumulating for more than two decades, for a number of reasons that will become clear, the evidence has not always seemed irrefutable. The general experimental strategies have been to show that destruction of all or part of the hippocampus, or of its projections to the hypothalamus (which include a projection from the subiculum to the CRF- and VP-containing paraventricular nucleus [93]), produce syndromes of adrenocortical hyperactivity, whereas electrical stimulation of the structure produces the opposite effect. In general, these results have been obtained, but they have become far more convincing in recent years because of two technical advancements. The first has been the use of more precise and delimited electrical stimulation. Early studies, stimulating at relatively high frequencies, produced conflicting results (11b,24,53,63,70,94,95) which weighed somewhat in favor of the hippocampus as an inhibitor of the HPA axis. More modern studies utilizing more discrete foci of stimulation have shown that all parts of the hippocampus, with the exception of the CA1 region, inhibit HPA secretion (23).

A second advancement has been the study of the HPA axis more proximally to the hippocampus. The earliest reports that hippocampal damage produced HPA hyperactivity predated widespread measurement of any of the HPA hormones themselves. Adrenal ascorbic acid depletion was instead the index of adrenal activity (26,56); this was obviously a most indirect measure. Subsequently, GCs themselves were measured, and supported the same general conclusions (33,52,57,85). However, the numerous steps between the hippocampus and the adrenal GC secretion are

all subject to their own   dynamic regulation (cf 54), and measurement
of GCs remained a very distal endpoint for these studies, one that can
easily obscure what is going on.

With time, ACTH could be measured reliably and sensitively, and
such studies demonstrated ACTH hypersecretion in the aftermath of
hippocampectomy. Importantly, this period of studies demonstrated that
the inhibition by the hippocampus was GC feedback inhibition, i.e.,
that the structure was mediating the inhibitory signal of circulating
GCs. This was demonstrated as follows: after hippocampectomy, ACTH
secretion was elevated, compared to controls. If both groups were then
adrenalectomized, ACTH secretion increased in both, but to equally
high concentrations (104). In other words, in the absence of a GC
negative-feedback signal, the presence or absence of the hippocampus
did not influence ACTH secretion.

The most direct endocrine demonstration of the inhibitory role of
the hippocampus would involve not the measure of ascorbic acid, GCs or
ACTH, but the direct measurement of ACTH-secretagogues, by cannulat-
ing the blood vessels in the hypothalamic portal system. This has
become possible only recently, due to the isolation and sequencing of
CRF, the recognition of the physiologic roles of the other secretagogues, and the development of sufficiently sensitive radioimmunoassays
and reliable cannulation techniques. Working in the laboratory in
which CRF was isolated, we first demonstrated that level sensitive
delayed GC feedback can occur at the level of the brain, primarily
expressed as the inhibition of stress-induced CRF secretion (72).
Recently, we have found that after cutting the fornix of rats, the
efficacy of such GC feedback inhibition is reduced, that hypersecretion
occurs at the level of the portal blood. Most interestingly, while
fornix cuts eventuate in only a moderate increase in CRF secretion,
the VP component of the signal to the pituitary is greatly augmented
(Sapolsky and Plotsky, in prep). Thus, these preliminary data give the
most direct support for the hippocampus as an inhibitor of the HPA
axis, and suggest that the hippocampus does so primarily via regulation of the more minor ACTH-secretagogues, rather than via CRF itself.

What form does the HPA hypersecretion take following hippocampal
damage? A variety have been reported. Basal concentrations of GCs
have been shown to be elevated, either throughout the circadian cycle,
or only at the circadian trough. The maximum plateau of GC secretion
during stress has also been reported to elevate (33,57,85). Two recent
reports examined whether hippocampal damage impaired the ability of
rats to inhibit GC secretion at the end of stress; both reported an
impaired capacity to appropriately terminate the stress response
(52,83). All of these incidences have been interpreted as representing
impaired sensitivity to feedback inhibition (87). Hippocampal damage
has been shown to be associated with a more explicit failure of such
sensitivity, as such rats have been shown to be DEX resistant (32).

In the primate, what little information is available supports a
similar role for the hippocampus. Electrical stimulation of the human
hippocampus inhibits GC concentrations (61,76). Furthermore, we have
recently found that fornix cuts in the macaque eventuate in cortisol
hypersecretion and a mild DEX resistance. Lesions of other regions,
including the amygdala, medial dorsal thalamus or mammillary bodies,
did not produce similar hypercortisolism (Sapolsky, Zola-Morgan and
Squire, unpublished).

A number of caveats are important in considering the hippocampus as an inhibitory site. First, its inhibitory input is not constant, but may occur only at certain points in the circadian cycle (35,66,104). Second, there is redundacy and plasticity in the system, in that the hippocampus does not appear to be the only such inhibitory site in the brain, and that other sites can assume a larger part of the role following damage to the hippocampus. Thus, there is recovery of function (35).

In summary, the hippocampus does appear to mediate GC feedback inhibitory signals to the hypothalamus. It should be emphasized, however, that its contribution to the HPA axis is limited. In other words, the extent of hypercortisolism after hippocampal damage is moderate. For those familiar with the pathophysiologic consequences of GC excess, even this moderate hypersecretion is meaningful. The adrenocortical axis is designed to convey rapid and small changes in information; such is only appropriate for a system conveying news of abrupt stressful emergencies. Under basal conditions, approximately 90% of circulating GCs are bound to transporting globulins, transcortin being the most important. Basally, transcortin is saturated, and it is the small free fraction of GCs which are biologically active at target tissues (103). Thus, a relatively small increase in GCs concentrations of, say, 10%, will essentially double the free fraction of the hormone reaching target sites. Furthermore, recent work has shown that GCs are far less the "all-or-none" permissive hormones they were traditionally considered, but rather have linear effects (20). Therefore, the relatively small GC hypersecretion following hippocampal damage can be physiologically, and pathophysiologically meaningful.

Receptor-mediated GC action at the hippocampus

Glucocorticoids, as steroid hormones, exert the bulk of their actions through their interaction with corticosteroid receptors. Such receptors are intracellular, rather than membrane bound, and the steroid hormone/receptor complex exerts its effects by interacting with genomic material to influence transcriptional events.

Within the brain, the hippocampus is considered as one of the prime target sites for GCs, because of its high concentrations of corticosteroid receptors. They are of two types, differing in their affinities for different endogenous and synthetic GCs, as well as their distribution (and likely functions) within the hippocampus (64).

It seemed obvious, given the dogma of steroid action, that if GCs exert some of their inhibitory effects upon the HPA axis via the hippocampus, that GC interaction with corticosteroid receptors in the hippocampus is an obligatory first step. Furthermore, it seemed conceivable that the hippocampus would become less sensitive to GCs, and would less faithfully transduce a GC signal into an inhibitory volley towards the hypothalamus, should it lose a significant portion of its corticosteroid receptors. We set about to test this idea-- would depletion of hippocampal corticosteroid receptors (without damaging the neurons of the hippocampus) produce HPA hypersecretion?

To do so, we developed two models of transient receptor depletion in the hippocampus. In both cases, the receptor loss was restricted, within the brain, to the hippocampus, and involved no damage to hippocampal neurons themselves. In the first model, we administered GCs to rats. Sustained exposure to high concentrations of GCs produces an autoregulatory decline in corticosteroid receptors. Of all brain structures, the hippocampus is preferentially sensitive to such "down-regulation" (84), such that it is possible to expose the rat to a GC regimen which will deplete the hippocampus of approximately 50% of such receptors without decreasing their concentrations elsewhere. In such receptor-depleted rats, a syndrome of HPA hypersecretion occurs. Specifically, rats were impaired in their capacity to terminate their stress-responses, continuing to secrete GCs after the end of stress when control subjects had terminated secretion. Upon cessation of GC administration, the receptor deficit spontaneously normalizes (84) and, importantly, the capacity to promptly terminate a stress-response returns at that time (85).

In the second model, we studied the Brattleboro rat, a strain congenitally lacking in VP. The peptide serves as an antidiuretic hormone in the pituitary, as a modulator of ACTH release, and as a neurotransmitter or neuromodulator in the brain. It appears that neural VP regulates concentrations of hippocampal corticosteroid receptors, as the Brattleboro rat has a depletion of approximately 50% of these receptors; administration of VP or of a centrally-acting VP analogue transiently corrects this deficit. The loss within the brain is exclusive to the hippocampal receptor population. We found that the Brattleboro rat hypersecretes GCs at the end of stress. Furthermore, normalization of hippocampal corticosteroid receptor concentrations with a VP analogue eliminates this hypersecretory defect. Finally, cessation of therapy with the VP analogue, which results in a progressive decline in receptor concentrations, is accompanied by a parallel re-emergence of the GC hypersecretion (85).

Thus, these studies indicate that hippocampal damage and, more subtly, mere loss of hippocampal corticosteroid receptors can produce HPA hypersecretion.

Hippocampal damage and hypercortisolism in the AD patient

Alzheimer's disease is a neurodegenerative disorder of unknown etiology whose main clinical features involves progressive loss of cognitive function. Neuropathologically, it is distinguished by neuronophagia, neurofibrillary tangles and amyloid plaques. Neuroanatomically, such degeneration is most pronounced in the nucleus basalis of Meynart in the basal forebrain, the hippocampus and overlying cortex (99). Neurochemically, it is the loss of cholinergic neurons arising in the nucleus basalis and projecting into the hippocampus and cortex which has attracted the most attention and is felt, by some, to underlie critically the cognitive impairments of the disease (19). In addition, other selective neurochemical losses (e.g., of somatostatin [21]) have been reported.

Does the hypercortisolism of some AD patients arise because of the hippocampal damage? We think this is possible, and is certainly in concordance with what is known about damage to the mammalian hippocampus. However, the studies outlined above have involved either destruction of the entire hippocampus, of at least half (i.e., dorsal or ventral), or complete severing of the fornical or septal projection. In comparison, the hippocampal neuronal damage in AD (while clearly severe enough to produce cognitive impairments) is far subtler. Will syndromes of HPA hypersecretion ensue with smaller extents of hippocampal damage?

This question has not yet been tested experimentally. However, an equivalent model occurs naturally in the rat. As a normal part of senescence in the male rat, hippocampal neurons are lost. This appears to occur progressively over the lifespan, and is most dramatic in the CA3 cellfield of the structure, such that by two years of age, perhaps 10-20% of neurons are lost in this region. As would be expected from a neuropathologic standpoint, such neuron loss is accompanied by microglial infiltration, presumably as a neuronophagic response to the ongoing neuron death (11,58,86). The aging hippocampus in the male rat thus normally sustains damage far more subtle than in cases of experimental lesion, and more akin, quantitatively, to what is observed in AD. Critically, such rats show a well-documented syndrome of HPA hypersecretion. Basal GC concentrations are elevated throughout the circadian cycle (22,59,83,85,98) (due to hypersecretion, rather than a change in the clearance rate of the hormone [83]). In addition, ACTH concentrations are increased (98). Measurement of CRF, VP or other secretagogues have not yet been performed. Furthermore, GCs are secreted excessively after the end of stress (47,83). Finally, aged male rats are resistant to feedback inhibition, whether induced by DEX (71) or by their naturally-occurring GC, corticosterone (88).

Thus, relatively more subtle hippocampal damage can be associated with DEX resistance and HPA hypersecretion, and supports the hypothesis that the hippocampal damage typical of AD may underlie the hypercortisolism of some sufferers. The data concerning the aging rat also help explain the previously mentioned pattern of DEX-resistance becoming more prevalent in older populations of AD patients. The aging human brain appears to undergo some loss of hippocampal neurons (1,4,62,65,67,91b). However, the aged healthy human is not hypercortisolemic; basal corisol secretion, circadian rhythmicity, clearance rate and DEX sensitivity are all intact (8,16,40,91,100-102). This suggests that hypercortisolism, while not obligatory among the normal aged or AD patient, is sub-clinical in both, and becomes far more penitrant when senescence and AD coincide.

What about additional sources of variability in DEX resistance in AD? In other words, what might explain the DEX resistance of one patient, and DEX sensitivity of another, both of the same age and extent of cognitive impairment? As a possibility, the two individuals may have similar extents of hippocampal damage, but the DEX resistant individual may have lost more of the neurons containing high concentrations of GC receptors. At this stage, essentially nothing is known of the individual cellular biology of hippocampal negative feedback, limiting the usefulness of these speculations.

Hippocampal corticosteroid receptor depletion and hypercortisolism in depression

The data presented in previous sections provide the following picture in the rat: during periods of sustained stress, GCs are secreted excessively. Through an autoregulatory mechanism, the high GC concentrations cause the number of corticosteroid receptors in the hippocampus to decrease. This is due to a decrease in the total number of such receptors in the neuron, rather than a mere ligand-induced occupation and translocation of receptors from the unoccupied pool (84). Such down-regulation most likely involves decreased synthesis of new receptors, rather than accelerated degradation of preexisting ones. Of all brain structures, such down-regulation occurs most readily in the hippocampus. On a teleological level, it makes some sense that the hippocampus, as a primary neural target tissue for

GCs, should be unduly sensitive to GC autoregulation. On a mechanistic level, it is not yet clear how this enhanced sensitivity is accomplished. With the down-regulatory loss of receptors, the hippocampus becomes less sensitive to circulating GCs and their feedback signal, and a syndrome of HPA hypersecretion ensues (85). When the prolonged stress and exposure to GCs abates, the concentration of receptors can normalize rapidly and normal HPA function returns.

Do these regulatory relations occur in the human? Nothing is known about steroid receptor autoregulation in the human brain. However, an indirect test supports the idea of parallelism in humans: sustained stress induces DEX resistance in primates. In one study of wild olive baboons, socially subordinate males (who are subject to the highest rates of social stressors) were found to have elevated basal concentrations of cortisol (81) and to be relatively DEX resistant, as compared to dominant individuals (82). (Because of the experimental constraints unique to studying wild primates, it was not possible to determine whether such subjects had absolute DEX resistance by the criteria of Carroll and colleagues [15]). Furthermore, when in the case of some males, rank rose, the hypercortisolism attenuated. In a supportive study, captive rhesus monkeys with the highest levels of behavioral arousal were found to be the most DEX resistant (50). Similar findings have emerged with human subjects. In one case that is, perhaps, most readily identified with by the readership, physicians were given DSTs during and after a period of sustained stress (preparation for a major case presentation at a clinical conference). Using a criteria for DEX resistance of 5 μg/dl, fully 44% of physicians were nonsuppressors during the period of stress. This occupational rigor appeared not to induce permanent damage, at least to this physiological system, as the incidence of resistance declined to 0% one week after the case presentation (7). Other reports (17) involving pre-surgical stress have reported similar rates of DEX resistance in non-depressed individuals.

Stress is recognized as a pre-disposing factor in depression (2). Is excessive stress necessary and sufficient to produce DEX resistance in a consequent depression? Certainly not, as borne out by the patterns of DEX resistant depressive populations. As with AD, there have to be interactions between a number of (in some cases, not yet measurable) factors: how much stress and GCs the person was exposed to; the concentration of hippocampal corticosteroid receptors prior to the stress; the sensitivity of such receptors to down-regulation; the threshold at which receptor depletion first impairs feedback inhibition. Some of these interactions can already be understood. As discussed, the aging primate hippocampus appears to lose neurons. Given the occurrence of corticosteroid receptors throughout the primate hippocampus (37), almost certainly the concentration of such receptors also declines with aging. However, this receptor loss is normally below threshold for impairing feedback inhibition; the healthy aged human is not hypercortisolemic. However, when age and depression coincide--with DEX resistance not being obligatory in either alone-- the incidence of DEX resistance increases dramatically. Thus, in older individuals, with hippocampal corticosteroid receptor concentrations already close to the threshold for feedback resistance, smaller amounts of stress may be needed to down-regulate receptor concentrations past the point of normal feedback sensitivity.

A recent study gives interesting, if indirect support to the idea that hippocampal dysfunction underlies DEX resistance in AD and depression. von Bardeleben and colleagues (6) administered DEX to healthy volunteers and examined which hypothalamic secretagogues could override the DEX suppression. They found that neither CRF nor VP alone could provoke cortisol secretion above the 5 μg/dl cut-off in the face of DEX suppression. However, a combination of the two overrode the inhibition. They argued that, to the extent that DEX resistance in the depressive appears to be a CNS phenomenon, it is likely to involve hypersecretion of both CRF and VP. In light of that conclusion, our preliminary findings that fornix section in the rat produces hypersecretion of both of these peptides is most suggestive.

How can these ideas be tested?

1. Determine whether in AD, DEX resistance is associated with more severe hippocampal damage upon post-mortem examination. Could such a trend be dissociated from severity of cortical damage?

2. Examine whether in AD, DEX resistance is associated with a loss of GC binding in the hippocampus, as measured by post-mortem receptor assays. Is this loss selective to the hippocampus? This approach has a number of difficulties:

   a. Individuals will have endogenous circulating GCs occupying these receptors at the time of death. This will make accurate determination of maximal binding capacity and affinity of receptors far more technically difficult.

   b. Comparisons should be made between AD patients who are DEX resistant versus DEX sensitive, yet who have similar basal GC concentrations. Should hippocampal GC receptor depletion be observed in DEX resistant individuals who are basally hypercortisolemic, one could argue that the depletion is a consequence of down-regulation, by the high GC concentrations, rather than a cause of the high concentrations.

   c. Post-mortems must be carried out as rapidly as is technically and ethically feasible, given the rapid post-mortem decay of these receptors. We have found that human brain tissue frozen three hours post-mortem already has barely measureable receptor concentrations (Sapolsky and Meaney, unpublished observations).

3. Examine whether in AD, DEX resistance is associated with loss of hippocampal GC binding, as measured with PET scanning with a tagged cortisol. Is a depletion specific to the HC? This approach has a number of advantages over receptor assays of post-mortem tissue, namely the avoidance of post-receptor decay, plus the ability to treat patients with a GC synthesis inhibitor (such as metyrapone) prior to PET scanning. This would avoid the problem of occupation of receptors by endogenous cortisol, and give more accurate measures of binding parameters. As with the post-mortem studies, the interpretively cleanest approach would be to compare individuals with similar basal cortisol values but who differ in being DEX sensitive or resistant. Finally, it is not clear if current PET scanning techniques will offer the resolution necessary for this study.

4. Determine whether in the depressive, DEX resistance is associated with decreased GC binding, exclusive to the hippocampus, as measured with PET scanning. All the same provisos and advantages as in point 3 hold.

5. In older depressives, if concentrations of hippocampal corticosteroid receptors are normatively declining towards the threshold for feedback insensitivity, less stress should have been

required to down-regulate receptor concentrations past that threshold than in young patients. Thus, the association between DEX resistance and a major predisposing stressor prior to the depression should be stronger in younger, than in older depressives.

6. Replicate the studies demonstrating that during periods of sustained stress, the incidence of DEX resistance in healthy individuals increases. Measure GC binding in the hippocampus with PET scanning before and during the period of stress. Examine whether those individuals with either the lowest absolute amounts of binding during stress, or who have undergone the greatest down-regulatory decline in binding are those who become most dramatically DEX resistant.

With the exception of point 5, which is an eminently feasable study, all of these are technically difficult experiments; perhaps they are merely thought experiments at this time. None address what we find to be a perplexing issue--the different, and potentially dissociated forms that HPA hypersecretion can take. Various forms of hippocampal damage have been reported to produce elevated basal, stress, or post-stress GC secretion, as well as feedback resistance. Yet, all these dysfunctions need not come in a package together. Likewise, depressive hypercortisolism can manifest itself as basal hypersecretion and/or feedback resistance, and again, both abnormalities need not occur in the same individual. At present, our understanding of how precisely the hippocampus works as a neuroendocrine transducer is so crude as to preclude any intelligent speculation on this issue.

In conclusion, hypercortisolism in AD and depression is of interest as a potentially informative marker about disease subtypes, as a wedge to understand other syndromes of GC excess, and to understand normative HPA function. It is our feeling that hippocampal dysfunction can underlie instances of hypercortisolism, particularly in AD and depression. Our own work in this area revolves around non-human subjects. It is our hope that this more than mildly speculative chapter might stimulate some tests of these ideas with regard to human neuroendocrine regulation.

References Cited

1. Anderson, J., Hubbard, B., Coghill, G. and Slidders, W. (1983) J. Neurol. Sci. 54:233.
2. Anisman, H., and Zacharko, R. (1982): Behav. Brain Sci. 5:89.
3. Asnis, G., Sachar, E., Halbreich, U., Nathan, R., Novacenko, H., and Ostrow, L. (1981): Psychosom. Med. 43:235.
4. Ball, M. (1977) Acta Neuropath. 37:111.
5. Balldin, J., Gottfries, C., Karlsson, I., Lindstedt, G., Langstrom G., and Walinder, J. (1983): Br. J. Psychiatry 143:277.
6. von Bardeleben, Holsboer, F., Stalla, G., and Muller, O. (1985): Life Sci. 37:1613.
7. Baumgartner, A., Graf, K., and Kurten, I. (1985): Biol. Psychiat. 20:675.
8. Blichert-Toft, M., and Hummer., L. (1976): J. Gerontol. 31:589.
9. Brown, W., and Qualls, C. (1981): Psychiat. Res. 4:115.
10. Brown, W., Johnston, R., and Mayfield, D. (1979): Am. J. Psychiat. 136:543.

11. Brizzee, K., and Ordy, J. (1979): Mech. Ageing Dev. 9:143.
11b. Bouille, C., and Bayle, J. (1973): Neuroendo 13:264.
12. Carnes, M., Smith, J., and Kalin, N. (1983): J. Am. Geriatric. Soc. 31:267.
13. Carnes, M., Smith, J., Kalin, N. (1983): Psychiatric Res. 9:337.
14. Carroll, B., Curtis, G., and Mendels, J. (1976): Arch. Gen. Psychiat. 33:1039.
15. Carroll, B., Feinberg, M., Greden, J. (1981): Arch. Gen. Psychiat. 38:15.
16. Cartlidge, N., Black, M., Hall, M., and Hall, R. (1970): Gerontol. Clin. 12:65.
17. Ceulemans, D., Westenberg, H., and van Praag, H. (1985): Psychiat. Res. 14:189.
18. Coryell W., and Zimmermann, M. (1983): Biol. Psychiat. 18:21.
19. Coyle, J., Price, D., and DeLong, M. (1983): Science 219:1184.
20. Dallman, M., Akana, S., Cascio, C., Darlington, D., Jacobson, L., and Levin, N. (1987): Rec. Prog. Horm. Res. 43:212.
21. Davies, P., Katzman, R., and Terry, R. (1980): Nature 288:279.
22. DeKosky, S., Scheff, S. and Cotman, C. (1984): Neuroendo. 38:33.
23. Dunn, J., and Orr, S. (1984): Exp. Brain Res. 54:1.
24. Dupont A., Bastarache, E., Endroczi, E., and Fortier, C. (1972): Can. J. Physiol. Pharmacol. 50:364.
25. Edwardson, J., and Bennett, G. (1974): Nature 251:425.
26. Endroczi, E., Lissak, K., Bohus, B., and Kovacs, S. (1959): Acta. Physiol. Acad. Sci. Hung. 16:17.
27. Evans, D., and Nemeroff, C. (1983): Biol. Psychiatry 18:505.
28. Evans, D., Burnett, G., and Nemeroff, C. (1983): Am. J. Psychiatry 140:586.
29. Fang, V., Tricou, B., Robertson, A., and Meltzer, H. (1981): Life Sci. 29:931.
30. Feldman, S., Chowers, I., and Conforti, N. (1973): Acta. Endo. 73:660.
31. Feldman, S., and Conforti, N. (1976): Horm. Res. 7:56.
32. Feldman, S., and Conforti, N. (1980): Neuroendo. 30:52.
33. Fendler, K., Karmos, G., Telegdy, M. (1961): Acta. Physiol. Scand. 20:293.
34. Fogel, B., Satel, S., and Levy, S. (1985): Psychiat. Res. 15:85.
35. Fischette, C., Komisurak, B., Ediner, H., Feder, H. and Siegel, A. (1980): Brain Res. 195:373.
36. Georgotas, A., Stokes, P., Krakowski, M., Fanelli, C., and Cooper, T. (1984): Biol. Psychiat. 19:685.
37. Gerlach, J., McEwen, B., and Pfaff, D. (1976): Brain Res. 103:603.
38. Gibbons, J. (1963): J. Psychosom. Res. 10:262.
39. Gold, P., Loriaux, L., Roy, A., Kling, M., Calabrese, J., Kellner, C., Nieman, L., Post, R., Pickar, D., Gallucci, W., Avgerinos, P., Paul, S., Oldfield, E., Cutler, G., and Chrousos, G. (1986): New Eng. J. Med. 314:1329.
40. Grad, B., Rosenberg, G., and Liberman, H. (1971): J. Gerontol. 26:351.
41. Greden, J., Kronfol, Z., Gardner, R., Feinberg, M., Mukhopadhyay, S., Albala, A., and Carroll, B. (1981): J. Affect. Disorders. 3:389.

42. Greden, J., Gardner, B., and King, D. (1983): Arch. Gen. Psychiat. 40:493.
43. Greenwald, B., Mathe, A., Mohs, R., Levy, M., Johns, C., and Davis, K. (1987): Am.J. Psychiat., in press.
44. Halbreich, U., Asnis, G., Zumoff, B., Nathan, R., and Shindledecker, R. (1984): Psychiat. Res. 13:221.
45. Hillhouse, E., and Jones, M. (1976): J. Endo. 71:21.
46. Holsboer, F., v Bardeleben, U., Gerken, A., Staller, G., and Muller, O. (1984): New Eng. J. Med. 311:1127.
47. Ida, Y., Tanaka, M., Tsuda, A., Kohno, Y.1, Hoaki, Y., Nakagawa, R., Iimori, K., and Nagasaki, N. (1984): Life Sci. 34:2357.
48. Jacobs, S., Mason, J., Kosten, T., Brown, S., and Ostfeld, A. (1984): Psychosom. Med. 46:213.
49. Jones, M., Hillhouse, E., and Burden, J. (1977): J. Endo. 73:405.
50. Kalin, N., Cohen, R., Kraemer, G., Risch, S., Shelton, S., cohen, M., McKinney, W., and Murphy, P. (1981): Neuroendo. 32:92.
51. Kalin, N., Weiler, S., and Shelton, S. (1982): Psychiat. Res. 7:87.
52. Kant, G., Meyerhoff, J., and Jarrard, L. (1984): Pharm. Biochem. Behav. 20:793.
53. Kawakami, M., Setko, K., Terasawa, E., Yoshida, K., Miyamoto, T., Sekiguchi, M., and Hattori, Y. (1968): Neuroendo 3:337.
54. Keller-Wood, M., Shinsako, J., and Dallman, M. (1983): Am. J. Physiol. 245:R53.
55. Keller-Wood, M., and Dallman, M. (1984): Endo. Rev. 5:1.
56. Kim, C., and Kim, C. (1961): Am. J. Physiol. 201:337.
57. Knigge K, and Hays, M. (1963): Proc. Soc. Exp. Biol. Med. 114:67.
58. Landfield, P., Rose, G., Sandles, L., Wohlstadter, T., and Lynch, G. (1977): J. Gerontol. 32:3.
59. Landfield, P., Waymire, J., and Lynch, G. (1978): Science 202:1098.
60. Lewis, D., Pfohl, B., Schlechte, J., and Coryell, W. (1984): Psychiat. Res. 13:213.
61. Mandell, A., Chapman, L., Rand, R., and Walter, R. (1963): Science 139:1212.
62. Mani, R., Lohr, J., and Jeste, D. (1986) Exp. Neurol. 94:29.
63. Mason, J. (1958): Endocrinol. 63:403.
64. McEwen, B., De Kloet, E., and Rostene, W. (1986): Physiol. Rev. in press.
65. Miller, A., Alston, R., Mountjoy, C., and Corsellis, J. (1984): Neuropath. Appl. Neurobiol. 10:123.
66. Moberg, G., Scapagnini, U., deGroot, J., and Ganong, W. (1971): Neuroendo. 7:11.
67. Mouritzen Dam, A. (1979): Neuropath. Appl. Nuerobiol. 4:249.
68. Nemeroff, C., Widerlov, E., Bissette, G., Walleus, H., Karlsson, I., Eklund, K., Kilts, C., Loosen, P. and Vale, W. (1984): Science 226:1342.
69. Nelson, W., Orr, W., Shane, S., and Stevenson, J. (1984): J. Clin. Psychiat. 45:120.
70. Nyakas, C., and Endroczi, E. (1970): Acta Physiol. Acad. Scient. Hung. 37:281.

71. Oxenkrug, G., McIntyre, I., Stanley, M. and Gershon, S. (1984): Biol. Psychiat. 19:413.

72. Plotsky, P., Otto, S., and Sapolsky, R. (1986): Endo. 119:1126.

73. Raskind, M., Peskind, E., and Rivard, M. (1982): Am. J. Psychiat. 139:1468.

74. Reus, V., Joseph, M., and Dallman, M. (1982): New Eng. J. Med. 306:23.

75. Rivier, C., and Plotsky, P. (1986): Ann. Rev. Physiol.

76. Rubin, R., Mandell, A., and Crandall, P. (1966): Science 153:767.

77. Rubinow, D., Post, R., Savard, R., and Gold P. (1984): Arch. Gen. Pschiat. 41:279.

78. Sachar, E., Hellman, L., Fukushima, D., and Gallagher, T. (1970): Arch. Gen. Psychiat. 23:289.

79. Sachar, E., Hellman, L., Roffwarg, H., Halpern, F., Fukushima, D., and Gallagher, T. (1973): Arch. Gen. Psychiat. 28:19.

80. Sachar, E., Asnis, G., Halbreich, U., Nathan, S., and Halpern, F. (1980): Psychiat. Clin. N. Am. 3:313.

81. Sapolsky, R. (1982): Horm. Behav. 15:279.

82. Sapolsky, R. (1983): Endo. 113:2263.

83. Sapolsky, R., Krey, L., and McEwen, B. (1983): Exp. Geront. 18:55.

84. Sapolsky, R., Krey, L., and McEwen, B. (1984): Endo. 114:287.

85. Sapolsky, R., Krey, L., and McEwen, B. (1984): Proc. Nat. Acad. Sci. (USA) 81:6174.

86. Sapolsky, R., Krey, L., McEwen, B. and Rainbow, T. (1984): J. Neurosci. 4:1479.

87. Sapolsky, R., Krey, L., and McEwen, B. (1986): Endocrine Revs. 7:284-301.

88. Sapolsky, R., Krey, L., and McEwen, B. (1986): Neurobio. Aging in press.

89. Schatzberg, A., Rothschild, A., Langlais, P.O., Bird, E., and Cole, J. (1985): J. Psychiat. Res. 19:57.

90. Schlesser, M., Winokur, G., and Sherman, B. (1980): Arch. Gen. Psychiat. 37:737.

91. Serio, M., Piolanti, P., Cappelli, G. (1969) Exp. Gerontol. 4:95.

91b. Shefer, V. (1977): Neurosci. Behav. Physiol. 8:236.

92. Sherman, B., Pfohl, B., and Winokur, G. (1984): Arch. Gen. Psychiat. 41:271.

93. Silverman, A., Hoffman, D., and Zimmerman, E. (1981): Brain Res. Bull. 6:47.

94. Smith, G., and Root, A. (1971): Neuroendo 8:235.

95. Slusher, M., and Hyde, J. (1961): Endo 68:773.

96. Spar, J., and Gerner, R. (1982): Am. J. Psychiat. 139:238.

97. Stokes, P., Stoll, P., Koslow, S., Maas, J., Davis, J., Swann, A., and Robins, E. (1984): Arch. Gen. Psychiat. 41:257.

98. Tang, G., and Phillips, R. (1978): J. Gerontol. 33:377.

99. Terry, R., and Katzman, R. (1983): Neurology 14:497.

100. Touitou, Y., Sulon, J., and Bogdan, A. (1983): J. Endo. 96:53.

101. Tourigny-Rivard, M., Raskind, M., and Rivard, D. (1981): Biol. Psychiat. 16:1177.

102. West, C., Brown, H., Simons, E., Carter, D., Kumagai, L., and Engelbert, E. (1961): J. Clin. Endo. Metab. 21:1197.

103. Westphal, U. (1971): Steroid-Protein interactions. Springe - Verlag, Berlin.

104. Wilson, M., Greer M., Greer, B., and Roberts, L. (1980): Brain Res. 197:433

105. Winokur, G., Pfohl, B., and Sherman, B. (1985): Biol. Psychiat. 20:751.

The studies described were made possible by support to the first author in the form of a pre-doctoral grant, from the National Institute on Aging, and a post-doctoral grant from the Life Sciences Research Foundation, of which the first author is a Mathers Fellow.

The Hypothalamic-Pituitary-Adrenal Axis:
Physiology, Pathophysiology, and Psychiatric
Implications, edited by A.F. Schatzberg and
C.B. Nemeroff. Raven Press, Ltd., New York
© 1988.

MULTIENDOCRINE ANALYSIS IN DEPRESSION

S. Craig Risch, M.D., David S. Janowsky, M.D.,
Lewis Judd, M.D., J.Christian Gillin, M.D.,
Miriam A. Mott, Jeffrey L. Rausch, M.D., and
Leighton Huey, M.D.

Psychiatry Service, San Diego Veterans
Administration Medical Center and
University of California, San Diego, M-003,
La Jolla, California,92093

ABSTRACT

Plasma concentrations of ACTH and prolactin were measured at 8 a.m. and 4 p.m. before and after the standard 1 mg overnight Dexamethasone Suppression Test (DST). Plasma concentrations of cortisol were measured at 8 a.m. and 4 p.m., and 11 p.m. before and after 1 mg dexamethasone. Dexamethasone suppressed plasma concentrations of ACTH, prolactin and cortisol in the subject group as a whole. "Cut Points" obtained using a Fisher's Exact Test identified plasma ACTH values at 8 a.m. baseline, 4 p.m. baseline and 8 a.m. post-dexamethasone and plasma prolactin values at all four times that significantly differentiated patients with bipolar depressive disorder and major depresssive disorder from other psychiatric patients. There were no cut points found at any of the six times for plasma levels of cortisol that significantly differentiated between these two diagnostic groups. A discriminant function analysis on baseline averages (8 a.m. and 4 p.m.) confirmed that ACTH and prolactin were excellent discriminators between these two diagnostic groups and that cortisol yielded little additional information in this subject group. Of interest in this subject population, basal (pre-dexamethasone) plasma concentrations were of more diagnostic information than post-dexamethasone values. These pilot findings suggest that monitoring plasma prolactin and ACTH concentrations before and after dexamethasone might increase the sensitivity and specificity of this laboratory test for depression.

INTRODUCTION

Adrenal cortisol hypersecretion, as well as flattened cortisol circadian periodicity, and failure to suppress plasma cortisol concentrations with the overnight 1 mg Dexamethasone Suppression Test (DST) occur in a significant number of endogenously depressed patients. Many (4-7,20-23) but not all (1,3,12,24) studies suggest that this neuroendocrine abnormality may be highly specific for melancholia. Many investigators also believe that this neuroendocrine abnormality may reflect limbic- hypothalamic-hypophyseal hyperactivity.

In this regard, Fang et al (9) and Reus et al (18) have reported that although dexamethasone-resistant depressed patients did not differ statistically from dexamethasone-sensitive depressed patients in baseline plasma ACTH concentrations, the dexamethasone-resistant depressed patients did have significantly higher post-dexamethasone plasma ACTH concentrations than did the dexamethasone-sensitive patients. Kalin et al (13) reported that dexamethasone-resistant patients have significantly higher pre- and post-dexamethasone plasma ACTH concentrations than do dexamethasone-sensitive patients. The data presented below also supports higher basal (pre-dexamethasone) plasma concentrations of ACTH in major depressive and bipolar depressed patients as compared with other groups of psychiatric patients.

Yerevanian et al (25) failed to demonstrate differences in ACTH plasma concentrations at 4 p.m. or 11 p.m. after dexamethasone in 19 normal volunteers, 10 depressed suppressors and 19 depressed nonsuppressors. However, they interpreted this lack of significant group differences as reflective of great inter-individual variation in adrenal sensitivity to circulating ACTH among the subjects within each group. In a later study, this group (26) reported that among 16 patients with major depressive disorder who were nonsuppressors on the DST upon hospital admission, that there was a significant reduction in plasma ACTH concentrations in patients whose DST normalized with clinical recovery, while ACTH levels remained high in the group that continued to be nonsuppressors.

These studies suggest that ACTH levels may be elevated in dexamethasone nonsuppressors and that monitoring plasma ACTH concentrations in the dexamethasone suppression test might be clinically useful.

In addition to suppressing plasma concentrations of cortisol and ACTH dexamethasone also suppresses plasma concentrations of prolactin. Meltzer et al (17) monitored the plasma prolactin response to dexamethasone in 52 psychiatric patients and reported a significant association between nonsuppression of plasma cortisol and prolactin after administration of dexamethasone.

In addition, basal prolactin levels have been reported as being elevated (15), unchanged (8,10), or low (2,14) in depressed subjects and an abnormal circadian secretion pattern for prolactin has been observed in depressed patients (11).

In a retrospective pilot study of 28 psychiatric subjects who had received the standard 1mg DST, we reported a significant group-time interaction when post-dexamethasone ACTH concentrations were compared between DST suppressors and nonsuppressors (19). In addition "cut-points" (Fisher Exact Test) of plasma prolactin at 0800 pre-dexamethasone and at 1600 post-dexamethasone and of plasma cortisol at 1600 pre-dexamethasone significantly differentiated patients with major depressive disorder and bipolar disorder from other psychiatric patients.

We now report a prospective study of the clinical utility of monitoring plasma ACTH and prolactin concentrations before and after dexamethasone in psychiatric inpatients in our Affective Disorders Unit at the San Diego Veterans Administration Medical Center (SDVAMC).

METHODS

These studies were conducted with the approval of the local human subjects committee. All subjects gave written, informed consent. All

subjects were male and there was no significant difference in age
composition among diagnostic groups. All subjects received a Schedule
of Affective Disorder and Schizophrenia (SADS) interview and Research
Diagnostic Criteria (RDC) diagnosis based on an interview by an
experienced diagnostician and collateral information obtained from
previous hospitalizations, medical records, and interviews with family
members. Diagnostic breakdown of the 46 subjects was as follows: major
depressive disorder (N = 22), bipolar depressive disorder (N = 10),
minor depressive disorder (N = 3) bipolar manic disorder (N = 3),
alcoholism (with and without secondary minor depression) (N = 3),
schizoaffective manic (N = 2), schizophrenic (N = 1), and RDC "other"
psychiatric disorder (N = 2), one patient with poly drug abuse, the
other patient with antisocial personality. One patient who had a
diagnosis of bipolar disorder mixed was classified as nondepressed
since, during his depressive periods he never met the criteria for major
depressive disorder. No subjects had received medications within 2
weeks prior to testing and alcoholic patients had been abstinent for at
least two months prior to study. No subjects were receiving medications
or had medical illnesses known to interfere with the DST or with plasma
concentrations of cortisol, ACTH or prolactin. All subjects were
inpatients on the Affective Disorders Clinical Research Unit of the San
Diego Veterans Administration Medical Center. All subjects were on the
same dietary regimen and were not receiving caffeinated beverages. All
subjects received the standard 1.0 mg Dexamethasone Suppression Test as
described by Carroll and colleagues (7). Blood samples for plasma
cortisol determinations were obtained at 8 a.m., 4 p.m., and 11 p.m.
before and after 1mg of dexamethasone. Blood samples for plasma ACTH
and prolactin determinations were only obtained at 8 a.m. and 4p.m.
before and after the DST because personnel were not available to process
samples properly for subsequent plasma prolactin and ACTH
determinations. Blood was collected in polypropyline EDTA tubes on ice
and promptly centrifuged at 12,350 g's for 20 minutes in a refrigerated
centrifuge and plasma was stored in a -80 C freezer until assayed
within 1-2 months. Ongoing quality control monitoring studies have
demonstrated the stability of these hormones collected and stored under
these conditions for up to and exceeding 6 months. Subjects whose
plasma cortisol concentrations equalled or exceeded 5 ug/dl at 8 a.m., 4
p.m., or 11 p.m. after dexamethasone were arbitrarily (see below)
classified as nonsuppressors.

ASSAY PROCEDURES

Plasma cortisol concentrations for the DSTs were performed in the
SDVAMC clinical laboratory using the Becton Dickinson I (125) cortisol
ARIA II System. The antibody is directed against cortisol-3-
carboxymetholoxime coupled to bovine thyroglobulin. Antibody
crossreactivities to aldosterone, testosterone, dihydrotestosterone,
progesterone, 17-α-OH progesterone, andostrene dione,
dehydro-epiandrosterone, 17-β-estradiol, and estriol are all less than
1.0%. Antibody crossreactivities are also as follows: cortiscosterone
10.6%, cortisone 12.6%, prednisone 19.3%, prednisolone 8.2%,
11-deoxycortisol 3.3%, and dexamethasone 1.6%. Assay sensitivity is 2
ug/dl and the upper limit of linearity is 64 ug/dl. The intra- assay
coefficient of variation is 4.8 - 5.9% and the interassay coefficient of
variation 4.9 - 8.6%. This assay has been validated by comparison of

identical samples of various cortisol concentrations with two other
RIAs in research laboratories.

Plasma ACTH measurements employed a sensitive RIA system developed
and described by Orth and co-workers. This well characterized antiserum has a higher affinity (KD > 1.07 x 10 - 12 M/liter) than any ACTH
antibody ever developed and is now commercially available from the IgG
Corporation of Nashville, Tennessee under Dr. Orth's direction. The
antiserum is of polyclonal origin yet it is specifically directed at the
steroidogenic NH_2-terminal (1-24) sequence of the whole (1-39) ACTH
molecule. Thus, it does not react with non-steroidogenic COOH-terminal
fragments of ACTH that can be found in circulating blood. The lack of
cross-reactivity with structurally and/or biosynthetically related
hormones (α-MSH, β -MSH, β -LPH and β -Endorphins allow the accurate
estimation of immunoreactive ACTH in as little as 100 ul of properly
prepared plasma. The optimized RIA system is capable of detecting as
little as 5 pg/ml of immunoreactive ACTH while maintaining a working
range of 0.5-75 pg/tube with 12.4 (% SD/X) throughout the standard
curve. The working standard ACTH reference preparation for this assay
is the synthetic human (1-39) sequence of adrenocorticotropin which is
available from Dr. Salvatore Raiti at the National Hormone and
Pituitary Program (NAIDDK). Samples were run in duplicate and intra-
assay variability is 3-5% and interassay variability is 4-8% at 80% and
20% B/BO.

Plasma prolactin (PRL) concentrations were determined in duplicate
using a RIA with reagents purchased from Calbiochem Corp. (La Jolla,
CA). The double antibody technique was used with human PRL for
iodination and standards, and with a rabbit anti-human PRL antibody.
The sensitivity of the assay was 0.8 ng/ml with interassay variation of
5% and interassay variation of 8%. Cross reactivities for the antibody
were: human TSH < 0.3%, human LH < 0.1%, human FSH < 1%, and human
GH < 0.3%.

STATISTICAL PROCEDURES

The data analysis was was performed by a doctorate level statistical
consultant and reviewed by two separate doctorate level statistical
consultants for accuracy and appropriateness of statistical methodology.
Of particular note, any subject without a complete data set was excluded
from a particular analysis. For example, if in an among subjects ACTH
analysis a 4 p.m. post-dexamethasone plasma concentration was not
available for a particular subject, i.e. blood not drawn, tube broken in
centrifuge, assay duplicate values not acceptable, and no further plasma
was available, then that subject was excluded from the ACTH analysis.
Thus, although 47 subjects were studied, the "N" of each analysis will
vary according to the availability of complete data sets for the
variable being analyzed.

Distributions of all three neuroendocrine assays were examined to
determine if they were sufficiently normal to perform parametric
statistics on raw values. With the exception of post-dexamethasone
cortisol values, it was determined that log transformation did not
sufficiently improve the shape of the distribution. Consequently, raw
values were used in analyses. Post-dexamethasone cortisol values were
analyzed nonparametrically.

Two-way between subjects ANOVAs were performed on 8 a.m. post-
dexamethasone minus 8 a.m. baseline and 4 p.m. post-dexamethasone minus

4 p.m. baseline change scores in order to assess the relationship of diagnosis and cortisol suppression to changes in ACTH and prolactin. Diagnosis was examined by assigning patients to "depressed" and "nondepressed" groups. Depressed patients were defined as those with RDS diagnoses of major depressive disorder (N=22) and bipolar depressive disorder (N=10). Nondepressed patients were defined as those with all other diagnoses listed above. The "depressed" patients had a mean age of 41.5 ± 8.5 year and mean Hamilton scores of 18.3 ± 7.1 and mean Beck scores of 23.5 ± 13.3 years and mean Hamilton scores 13.3 ± 8.0 and mean Beck scores of 16.1 ± 13.5.

Patients were also assigned to groups according to whether or not cortisol levels were suppressed by dexamethasone. Dexamethasone nonsuppression was defined by post-dexamethasone cortisol levels greater than or equal to 5.0 ug/dl at 8 a.m., 4 p.m., or 11 p.m. post 1.0 mg dexamethasone. Post-dexamethasone criteria of less than or equal to 4.0 ug/dl and greater than or equal to 6.0 ug/dl were also evaluated with similar results.

Four factor Mixed ANOVAs were utilized to determine the effects and interactions between diagnosis, cortisol suppression, day (baseline vs. post-dexamethasone) and time of day in ACTH and prolactin levels.

A computerized program using a Fisher's Exact Test was utilized to determine cutpoints that differentiated significantly between the two diagnostic groups (depressed vs. nondepressed).

A discriminant function analysis was calculated on baseline average (8 a.m. and 4 p.m.) of ACTH, prolactin, and cortisol to determine the maximum discriminant ability of combinations of neuroendocrine values.

Spearman's Rank Order correlation was used to determine the degree of association between the neuroendocrine values and change scores (baseline minus postdexamethasone plasma concentrations of the same time of day).

RESULTS

Only 11 of 32 depressed patients met DSM-III criteria for melancholia, and 22 of the 32 patients met RDC criteria for endogenous depression. Of the nine depressed patients who did not suppress cortisol, the breakdown of subtypes was as follows: four met criteria for both melancholia and endogenous depression, one met criteria for endogenous only, two met criteria for probable endogenous only, and two did not meet criteria for either subtype. Of the four nondepressed cortisol nonsuppressors, two were diagnosed as Bipolar I, manic, and two were diagnosed as having minor depressive disorder.

Mean plasma concentrations of ACTH, prolactin, and cortisol before and after standard 1 mg Dexamethasone Suppression Test are presented in TABLE 1.

TABLE 1. _Plasma concentrations of ACTH, prolactin, and cortisol for two diagnostic categories_

	PRE-DEXAMETHASONE		
ACTH (pg/ml)	0800	1600	2300
Depressed (N=23)	32.27±4.18	26.33±2.96	- - - -
Non-depressed (N=13)	22.18±2.07	17.52+1.63	- - - -

PRE-DEXAMETHASONE

PROLACTIN (ng/ml)

Depressed (N=25)	17.00+1.00	15.66+1.11	- - - -
Non-depressed (N=13)	22.01+2.74	19.98+2.87	- - - -

CORTISOL (ug/dl)

Depressed (N=23)	15.76+1.15	10.12+0.86	4.90+0.55
Non-depressed (N=14)	17.76+1.24	10.65+1.12	7.56+2.54

POST-DEXAMETHASONE

ACTH (pg/ml)	0800	1600	2300
Depressed (N=23)	12.00+1.58	12.18+1.81	- - - -
Non-depressed (N=23)	12.28+2.50	11.64+1.43	- - - -

PROLACTIN (ng/ml)

Depressed (N=25)	13.04+0.78	14.73+1.29	- - - -
Non-depressed (N=13)	17.55+2.78	18.96+2.63	- - - -

CORTISOL (ug/dl)

Depressed (N=23)	2.27+0.20	2.47+0.27	2.71+0.31
Non-depressed (N=23)	3.96+1.15	3.79+0.95	3.07+0.50

ACTH

There were no significant main effects or interactions between diagnosis and cortisol suppression for 8 a.m. ACTH change scores. (8 a.m. post-dexamethasone minus 8 a.m. baseline values), such that the change in ACTH at 8 a.m. between days was not significantly different between either depressed and nondepressed patients or cortisol suppressors or nonsuppressors.

There was a trend toward a diagnosis effect on 4 p.m. ACTH change scores (post-dexamethasone minus baseline) between depressed and nondepressed patients ($F(1,34) = 3.28$, p = .0769). The difference appears to be attributable to the higher ACTH concentrations in the depressed patients at baseline (FIG. I). Analysis of diagnosis effect on baseline ACTH values (8 a.m. and 4 p.m.) revealed significantly higher ACTH levels ($F(1,36) = 5.38$, p .05) in depressed patients in comparison to nondepressed patients.

There were also a significant main effect of cortisol suppression on 4 p.m. ACTH change scores ($F(1,34) = 4.587$, p .05) (TABLE 2). This appears to be due to the fact that cortisol suppressors had higher levels of ACTH at 4 p.m. baseline, but dropped more sharply to lower at 4 p.m. post-dexamethasone than did cortisol nonsuppressors (FIG. II). There was no significant diagnosis by suppression interaction for 4 p.m. change scores.

FIG. I   Plasma concentrations of ACTH (pg/ml), cortisol (ug/dl), and prolactin (ng/ml), before and after the standard 1 mg. Dexamethasone Suppression Test in depressed and nondepressed patients.

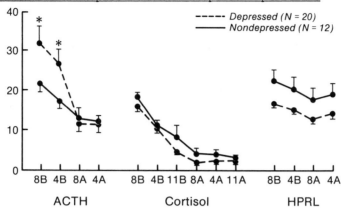

TABLE 2.   Significant effects and interactions for change in ACTH and Prolactin, before and after dexamethasone at 1600 hrs.

ACTH (pg/ml)
Main Effect of Cortisol Suppression--F(1,34) = 4.59, p = 0.04

Group	Mean ± SEM	N
Suppressors	-13.15 +2.32	28
Nonsuppressors	- 4.01 +2.01	10

Prolactin (ng/ml)
Diagnosis X Suppression Interaction--F(1,37) = 4.81, p = 0.03

	Diagnosis			
Group	Depressed	N	Nondepressed	N
Suppressors	-0.89 + 0.76	21	-3.06 + 2.15	9
Nonsuppressors	-1.11 + 0.85	7	3.55 + 1.93	

FIG. II   Plasma concentrations of ACTH (pg/ml), cortisol (ug/dl), and prolactin (ng/ml), before and after the standard 1 mg.Dexamethasone Suppression Test in cortisol suppressors (values less than 5 ug/dl) and nonsuppressors (values greater than or equal to 5 ug/dl).

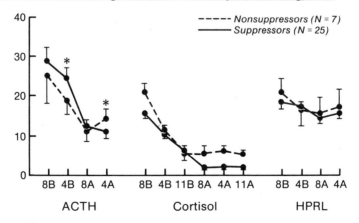

For ACTH, the four-factor Mixed ANOVA yielded the expected significant main effects of day (dexamethasone suppressed ACTH levels) and the ACTH levels were lower at 4 p.m. than 8 a.m.   There were also a significant day by time interaction (TABLE 3).   Tukey's post hoc test for unconfounded interactions showed this was due to the decrease from 8 a.m. to 4 p.m. on baseline as well as differences from pre- to post-dexamethasone for 8 a.m. and 4 p.m.   There were no other significant main effects or interactions.

TABLE 3. <u>Diagnosis by suppression by day by time Analysis of Variance--Main effects and interactions for ACTH and Prolactin</u>

<u>ACTH</u> (pg/ml)

1) Main Effect of Day

<u>Day</u>	<u>N</u>	<u>X $\pm$ SEM</u>	<u>F(df $=$ 1,32)</u>	<u>p-value</u>
Pre-dexamethasone	36	25.89 + 2.23	41.96	.0000
Post-dexamethasone	36	12.04 + 1.21		

2) Main Effect of Time

<u>Time</u>	<u>N</u>	<u>X $\pm$ SEM</u>	<u>F(df $=$ 1,32)</u>	<u>p-value</u>
0800	36	20.36 + 1.68	4.59	.0398
1600	36	17.57 + 1.41		

3) Day by Time Interaction

<u>Day</u>	<u>N</u>	<u>0800</u> <u>X $\pm$ SEM</u>	<u>N</u>	<u>1600</u> <u>X $\pm$ SEM</u>	<u>F(1,32)</u>	<u>p-value</u>
Pre-dexa- methasone	36	28.62 + 2.87	36	23.15 + 2.09	5.22	.0291
Post-dexa- methasone	36	12.10 + 1.33	36	11.99 + 1.25		

<u>PROLACTIN</u> (ng/ml)

1) Main Effect of Day

<u>Day</u>	<u>N</u>	<u>X $\pm$ SEM</u>	<u>F(df $=$ 1,32)</u>	<u>p-value</u>
Pre-dexamethasone	38	17.93 + 1.15	23.06	.0000
Post-dexamthasone	38	15.38 + 1.15		

2) Day by Time Interaction

<u>Day</u>	<u>N</u>	<u>0800</u> <u>X $\pm$ SEM</u>	<u>N</u>	<u>1600</u> <u>X $\pm$ SEM</u>	<u>F(1,34)</u>	<u>p-value</u>
Pre-dexa- methasone	38	18.71 + 1.19	38	17.14 + 1.25	16.22	.0003
Post-dexa- methasone	38	14.58 + 1.11	38	16.18 + 1.26		

3)Day by Suppression by Diagnosis Interaction

Nondepressed	N	Suppressors	N	Nonsuppressors	F(1,34)	p-value
Pre-dexa-methasone	9	21.19 + 2.85	4	20.55 + 6.60	4.78	.0358
Post-dexa-methasone	9	17.27 + 2.47	4	20.49 + 7.26		

Depressed						
Pre-dexa-methasone	20	16.70 + 1.17	5	14.86 + 1.13		
Post-dexa-	20	14.60 + 1.16	5	11.03 + 0.95		

PROLACTIN (ng/ml)--1600 Pre-Dexamethasone

	24.5	24.5	p-value		
Depressed	27	2	.0213	Sensitivity	= 93.10%
Nondepressed	8	5		Specificity	= 38.46%
				PV+	= 77.14%
				PV-	= 71.43%
				Efficiency	= 76.19%

PROLACTIN (ng/ml)---0800-Dexamethasone

	23.6	23.6	p-value		
Depressed	31	0	.300	Sensitivity	= 100.0%
Nondepressed	12	3		Specificity	= 20.00%
				PV+	= 72.09%
				PV-	= 100.0%
				Efficiency	= 73.91%

PROLACTIN (ng/ml)--1600 Post-Dexamethasone

	13.1	13.1	p-value		
Depressed	18	13	.01158	Sensitivity	= 58.06%
Nondepressed	3	12		Specificity	= 80.00%
				PV+	= 85.71%
				PV-	= 48.00%
				Efficiency	= 65.22%

Sensitivity = true positive rate = % depressed patients with abnormal
            values.
Specificity = true negative rate = % nondepressed patients with normal
            values
PV+   = predictive value of abnormal test = % of abnormal values
            that are in depressed patients, at the stated prevalence
            of depression.
PV-   = predictive value of a normal test = % of normal values
            that are in nondepressed patients.
Efficiency = % of all results that are true results, whether depressed
            or nondepressed patients.

The Fisher's Exact test identified several cutpoints for ACTH values at 8 a.m. baseline, 4 p.m. baseline, and 8 a.m. post-dexamethasone that discriminated significantly between depressed and nondepressed patients. The cutpoint that was the best discriminator for each time is presented in TABLE 4.

TABLE 4. Cutpoints Obtained Using a Fisher's Exact Test That Differentiate Significantly Between Depressed and Nondepressed Patients.

	ACTH (pg/ml)--0800		Pre-Dexamethasone	
	33.0	33.0	p-value	
Depressed	16	10	.0277	Sensitivity = 38.46%
Nondepressed	14	1		Specificity = 93.33%
				PV+ = 90.91%
				PV- = 46.67
				Efficiency = 41.5%

	ACTH (pg/ml)--1600		Pre-Dexamethasone	
	24.5	24.5	p-value	
Depressed	16	12	.0039	Sensitivity = 42.86%
Nondepressed	13	0		Specificity = 100.0%
				PV+ = 100.0%
				PV- = 44.83%
				Efficiency = 39.0%

	ACTH (pg/ml)--0800		Post-Dexamethasone	
	11.0	11.0	p-value	
Depressed	12	19	.0287	Sensitivity = 61.29%
Nondepressed	11	4		Specificity = 73.33%
				PV+ = 82.61%
				PV- = 47.83%
				Efficiency = 38.4%

	PROLACTIN (ng/ml)--0800		Pre-Dexamethasone	
	21.7	21.7	p-value	
Depressed	24	2	.0188	Sensitivity = 92.31%
Nondepressed	9	6		Specificity = 40.00%
				PV+ =
72.73%				
				PV- =
75.00%				
				Efficiency = 73.17%

PROLACTIN

There were no significant main effects or interactions between diagnosis and cortisol suppression for 8 a.m. prolactin change scores (8 a.m. post-dexamethasone minus 8 a.m. baseline values), such that the change in prolactin at 8 a.m. between days was not significantly different between either depressed and nondepressed patients or cortisol suppressors or nonsuppressors.

There were also no significant main effects of diagnosis or cortisol suppression for 4 pm. prolactin change scores (4 p.m. post-dexamethasone minus 4 p.m. baseline). There was a significant diagnosis by cortisol suppression interaction ($F(1,27) = 4.810$, $p < .05$) (TABLE 2). Tukey's post hoc test for unconfounded interactions showed the significant interaction was due to the difference between nondepressed cortisol suppressors and nondepressed cortisol nonsuppressors. Among the nonsuppressed group, patients who suppressed cortisol also had suppression of prolactin levels while cortisol nonsuppressors did not suppress prolactin, a relationship which was not apparent in the depressed group.

For prolactin, the four-factor Mixed ANOVA yielded a significant main effect of day (dexamethasone suppressed prolactin), and a significant day by time interaction (TABLE 3). Tukey's post hoc test for unconfounded interactions showed this overall significance to be due to the decrease of 8 a.m. to 4 p.m. on baseline, as well as the increase from 8 a.m. to 4 p.m. post-dexamethasone. Additionally, 8 a.m. levels of prolactin decreased significantly from pre- to post-dexamethasone. There was no significant main effect of time (8 a.m. to 4 p.m.). There was a trend toward a significant relationship between diagnosis and prolactin ($F(1,34) = 4.009$, $p = .0533$), with the depressed group having lower mean prolactin values (mean +/-SEM = 15.11 +/-0.95, N = 25 than the nondepressed group (mean +/- SEM = 19.63 +/- 2.61 N, = 13).

Additionally, there was a significant three-way day by cortisol suppression by diagnosis interaction for prolactin ($F(1,33) = 3.778$, $p < .05$) (TABLE 3). Simple interactions of diagnosis by day as well as cortisol suppression by day were calculated post hoc to locate the sources of the overall significant interaction. Neither of these simple interactions was significant. Thus, there was no significant diagnostic influence on dexamethasone effects among cortisol suppressors or nonsupressors considered independently. However, as can be seen in TABLE 3, the changes in prolactin for cortisol suppressors and nonsuppressors across day were in opposite directions for the depressed and nondepressed groups, thus resulting in the significant three-way interaction. Specifically, in the nondepressed group, prolactin levels in cortisol suppressors changed more from after dexamethasone than in cortisol nonsuppressors. However, in the depressed group, cortisol suppressors changed less from pre- to post-dexamethasone than cortisol nonsuppressors.

Fisher's Exact Test identified several cutpoints at all four times that could significantly discriminate between depressed and nondepressed patients. The cutpoint that was the best discriminator for each time is presented in TABLE 4.

CORTISOL

Post-dexamethasone cortisol values were not normally distributed and were analyzed nonparametrically, since values for many of the subjects were below the lower limit of sensitivity of the assay (2.0 ug/dl). The baseline cortisol values were analyzed using a two factor mixed analysis of variance to assess significant effects of diagnosis and time. Though baseline cortisol values showed the expected decrease over time from 8 a.m. to 11 p.m. ($F(2,70) = 45.447$, $p < .0001$), the main diagnosis effect and the diagnosis by time interaction were not significant.

Post-dexamethasone cortisol values were analyzed using Fisher's Exact Test. Subjects were dichotomized by cortisol levels (< 5.0 ug/dl vs. $\geq$ 5.0 ug/dl at any post-dexamethasone time) and by diagnosis (depressed versus nondepressed). The frequency of depressed nonsuppressors did not differ significantly from nondepressed nonsuppressors (TABLE 5).

TABLE 5. <u>Contingency table and Fisher's Exact Test for post-dexamethasone cortisol values</u>

	<u>Suppressors</u>	<u>Nonsuppressors*</u>	<u>Fisher's Exact p</u>
Depressed	23	9	.6037 (n/s)
Nondepressed	11	4	

Re DST:

Sensitivity	=	28.1%
Specificity	=	73.3%
PV+	=	69.23%
PV-	=	32.35%
Efficiency	=	42.55%

*Nonsuppressors are defined as subjects obtaining a cortisol value of 5.0 ug/dl or greater at any post-dexamethasone time point (0800, 1600 or 2300).

Additionally, baseline and post-dexamethasone cortisol levels were examined using the computerized Fisher's Exact Test to identify any cutpoint that would differentiate significantly between the two diagnostic groups. There were no cutpoints found at any time point that discriminated significantly between depressed and nondepressed patients.

DISCRIMINANT FUNCTION ANALYSIS

A discriminant function analysis was performed on baseline averages (8 a.m. and 4 p.m. of all three neuroendocrine measurements to determine relative diagnostic classification ability. The multi-variate analysis yielded a statistically significant difference between the two diagnostic groups. Univariate results illustrate this finding in TABLE 6. Standardized discriminant function coefficients show that either baseline ACTH or prolactin are excellent discriminators between diagnostic groups, and that baseline cortisol poorly discriminates. TABLE 6 also shows the classification results of the discriminant function analysis, indicating predicted vs. actual group membership.

TABLE 6. <u>Discriminant Function results for baseline average (0800 and 1600) of ACTH, Prolactin, and Cortisol.</u>

<u>Group</u> <u>Means</u>

		<u>ACTH X + SEM</u>	<u>PROLACTIN X + SEM</u>	<u>CORTISOL X + SEM</u>
Nondepressed	13	19.85 + 1.63	21.00 +2.67	13.96+1.13
Depressed	22	30.14 + 3.31	15.64 +0.74	13.46 + 0.92

<u>Univariate</u> <u>Results</u> (df = 1,33)

VARIABLE	WILKS' LAMBDA	EQUIVALENT F	P-VALUE
ACTH baseline average (pg/ml)	.86366	5.210	.0290
Prolactin baseline average (ng/ml)	.85314	5.681	.0231
Cortisol baseline average (ug/dl)	.99658	0.113	.7387

Multivariate Results (df = 3)
Wilks' Lambda =   .73508
Chi Squared   = 9.6947, p = .0213

Standardized Discriminant Function Coefficients
ACTH baseline average   = -0.72159
Prolactin baseline average = 0.72868
Cortisol baseline average = 0.19276

Classification Results

		PREDICTED GROUP	
ACTUAL GROUP	N	NONDEPRESSED	DEPRESSED
Nondepressed	13	9 (69.2%)	4 (30.8%)
Depressed	22	6 (27.3%)	16 (72.7%)

Percent of grouped cases correctly classified = 71.43%

CORRELATIONS

Correlations were calculated using Spearman's Rank Order Correlation Coefficient on pre- and post-dexamethasone levels of ACTH, prolactin, and cortisol, as well as on 8 a.m. and 4 p.m. change scores for ACTH and prolactin. Although some correlations were statistically significant, all were small ($r \leq 0.3$) and of doubtful biological or clinical significance. Similarly, post-dexamethasone, 1600 cortisol values correlated only weakly with age ($r = .32$, $p < .05$) and post-dexamethasone 0800 cortisol levels correlated weakly with Hamilton Score ($r = .31$, $p < .05$). No other time points of any neuroendocrine plasma levels correlated with age. Hamilton or Beck scores.

DISCUSSION

The present results parallel other reports that bipolar depressed and major depressive disorder patients have significant abnormalities of plasma cortisol ACTH and in some studies (2) low plasma concentrations of prolactin. Specifically, in our sample, abnormalities of ACTH suppression by dexamethasone were noted, and 4 p.m. pre-dexamethasone ACTH levels were better discriminators of bipolar depressed and major depressive disorder patients from other types of patients than plasma cortisol concentrations. Matthews and colleagues (19) have similarly reported that post-dexamethasone plasma concentrations of anterior pituitary -endorphin-like immunoreactivity were better nosological discriminators than post-dexamethasone cortisol levels. These results also suggest that the abnormality in adrenal cortisol hypersecretion widely noted in depressed patients may represent, at least in part, dysfunction at the pituitary or even more central levels. In this patient sample, pre- or post-dexamethasone plasma cortisol concentrations did not prove useful diagnostic discriminators for major depressive disorder and bipolar depressive patients, while low basal plasma prolactin and high basal plasma ACTH concentrations were powerful markers for nosological classification. Furthermore, a discriminant function analysis (see above) using both basal plasma prolactin and ACTH concentrations provided the most powerful means of differentiating patients with major depressive disorder and bipolar disorder from other

patients. Given the relative infrequency of depressed subjects with
melancholia in our sample (as noted above), it may be that derangements
of anterior pituitary prolactin and ACTH secretion in this patient
sample represents a more subtle indicator of
hypothalamic-pituitary-adrenal axis dysfunction than do pre- or
post-dexamethasone plasma cortisol concentration.

These results are not in any way in apparent conflict with the
previously reported (7) utility of monitoring post-dexamethasone plasma
cortisol concentrations in melancholic patients. As noted above a
relatively few of our depressed subjects had melancholia or abnormal
DSTs. However, the "depressed" subjects in our study population
(arbitrarily defined in this study as RDC major depression or bipolar
depression) while perhaps not as severely or "purely" depressed as
melancholic subjects, do in fact appear to have neuroendocrine
abnormalities of diagnostic importance.

In this subject population, the depressed patient's neuroendocrine
abnormalities were more manifest at baseline, i.e. pre-dexamethasone
than after dexamethasone. Dr. Stanley Watson (personal communication)
has hypothesized that since the depressed subjects in this study tended
not to have significantly higher basal pre-dexamethasone plasma cortisol
concentrations than the comparison group of psychiatric subjects, it is
conceivable that the elevated "basal" predexamethasone plasma ACTH
concentrations observed in the "depressed" subjects in this study result
from a relative lack of negative feedback by cortisol which may occur in
more severely depressed, cortisol hypersecreting, melancholic subjects.
It may be that monitoring both basal pre-dexamethasone and post-
dexamethasone plasma cortisol and ACTH concentrations in the DST might
identify more RDC depressed subjects, with post-dexamethasone
neuroendocrine abnormalities being more manifest in patients with
melancholia and pre-dexamethasone abnormalities being more manifest in
those depressed subjects without melancholia.

In this subject group as a whole, we were unable to demonstrate
significant nonsuppressability of plasma prolactin concentrations
accompanying cortisol dexamethasone nonsuppressors. However, our data
indicate a significant diagnostic difference in the way cortisol
suppressors and nonsuppressors change from following dexamethasone such
that in the nondepressed group, prolactin levels for cortisol
nonsuppressors did not change as much in response to dexamethasone as
did cortisol nonsuppressors in the depressed group.   Additionally,
prolactin levels in our sample tended to be lower before and after
dexamethasone in bipolar depressed and major depressive disorder
patients than other nosological types of patients, as has been reported
by others (2,14).

As discussed above, since our depressed subjects tended not to have
elevated baseline predexamethasone cortisol plasma concentrations
commonly observed in melancholic subjects, this might account for the
absence of elevated basal predexamethasone prolactin and the absence of
subsequent dexamethasone relative nonsuppressability of prolactin
observed in the study of Meltzer and colleagues (17) since the subjects
in that study appeared more severely depressed, more frequently
melancholic,and more commonly DST nonsuppressors (17). It may be that
plasma prolactin concentrations, like plasma ACTH and cortisol may vary
along a continuum reflecting severity.

These results need replication with much larger sample sizes, but
suggest to us that concomitant measurement of pre-and post-dexamethasone

plasma ACTH and prolacting (and B-endorphin-like Immunoreactivity in a previous study, Matthews et al (16) may be of clinical utility in improving the sensitivity and specificity of the DST, and in understanding neuroendocrine dysfunction in depression.

ACKNOWLEDGMENTS

This work was supported, in part, by the San Diego Veterans Administration Medical Center, and grants MH 00393, MH 39113, and MH 30914.

REFERENCES

1. Amsterdam, J.D., Winokur, A., Caroff, S.N., and Conn,J. (1982): Am. J. Psychiatr., 139:287-291.
2. Asnis, G.M., Nathan, R.S., Halbreich, U., Halpern, F.S., and Sachar, E.J. (1980): Am J. Psychiatr., 137:1117-1118.
3. Berger, M., Doerr, P., Lund, T., Bronisch, and T., v. Zerssen, F. (1982): Biol. Psychiat., 17:1217-1242.
4. Brown, W.A., Johnston, R., and Mayfield, D. (1979): Am. J. Psychiatr. 136:543-548.
5. Carroll, B.J., Curtis, G.C., and Mendels, J. (1976): Arch. Gen. Psychiat., 33:1039-1044.
6. Carroll, B.J., Curtis, G.C., and Mendels, J. (1976): Arch. Gen. Psychiat., 33:1051-1058.
7. Carroll, B.J., Feinberg, M., Greden, J.F., Tarika, J., Albala, A.A., Haskett, R.F. , James, N.M., Kronfol, Z., Lohr, N., Steiner, M., de Vigne, J.P., and Young, E. (1981):Arch. Gen. Psychiat., 38:15-22
8. Ehrensing, R.H., Kostin, A.J., Schach, D.S., Friesen, H.G., Vargas, J.R., and Schally, A.V. (1974): Am. J. Psychiatr., 131:714-718.
9. Fang, V.S., Tricou, B.J., Robertson, A., and Meltzer, H.Y. (1981): Life Sci., 29:931-938.
10. Gregoire, E., Brauman, H., DeBuch, H., and Corvilain, V. (1977): Psychoneuroendocrinology, 2:303-312.
11. Halbreich, U., Guinhaus, L., and Ben-David, M. (1979):Arch. Gen. Psychiatr., 36:1183-1188.
12. Holsboer, F., Bender, W., Benkert, O., Klein, H.E., and Schmauss, M. (1980): The Lancet i, 706.
13. Kalin, N.H., Weiler, S.J., and Shelton, S.E. (1982): Psychiatry Research, 7:87-91.
14. Linkowski, P., Brauman, H., and Mendlewicz, J. (1980): Psychiatry Research, 3:265-271.
15. Maeda, K., Kato, Y., Ohgo, S., Chichara, K., Yoshimoto, Y., Yamaguchi, N., Kuromaura, S., and Imura, H. (1975): J. Clin. Endo. Metab.,40:501-50
16. Matthews, J., Akil, H., Greden, J., and Watson, S. (1982):Life Sci., 31:1867-1870.
17. Meltzer, H.Y., Fang, V.S., Tricou, B.J., Robertson, A., and Piyaka, S.K. (1982): Am. J. Psychiat., 139:763- 768.
18. Reus, V.I., Joseph, M.S., and Dallman, M.F. (1982):New England J.Med., 306:238-239
19. Risch, S.C., Janowsky, D.S., Gillin, J.C., Mott, M. and Huey, L.Y. (in press): In: Clinical and Pharmacological Studies in Psychiatric Disorders, edited by G.D. Burrow and Trevor R.Norman.

20. Sachar, E.J. Neuroendocrine dysfunction in depressive illness
    (1976):Ann. Rev. Med., 27:389.
21. Sachar, E.J., Asnis, G., Nathan, R.S., Halbreich, U., Tabrizi,M.A.,
    and Halpern, F.S. (1980): Arch. Gen. Psychiat., 37:755-757.
22. Schlesser, M.A., Winokur, G., and Sherman, B.M. (1980): Arch. Gen.
    Psychiatry Psychiatr., 37:737-743.
23. Stokes, P.E., Pick, G.R., Stoll, P.M., and Nunn, W.D. (1975): J.
    Psychiat. Res., 12:271-282.
24. Stokes, P.E., Stoll, P.M., Koslow, S.H., Maas,J.W.,Davis,
    J.M., Swann, A.C., and Robins, E. (1984): Arch. Gen. Psychiatr.,
    Psychiat.,41:257-267.
25. Yerevanian, B.I. and Woolf, P.O. (1983):Psychiatry Research,9:45-51.
26. Yerevanian, B.I., Woolf, P.O., and Iker, H.P. (1983):Psychiatry
    Research, 10:175- 181.

The Hypothalamic-Pituitary-Adrenal Axis:
Physiology, Pathophysiology, and Psychiatric
Implications, edited by A.F. Schatzberg and
C.B. Nemeroff. Raven Press, Ltd., New York
© 1988.

BIOCHEMICAL AND NEUROENDOCRINE STUDIES
IN PSYCHOTIC AND NONPSYCHOTIC DEPRESSIONS

Anthony J. Rothschild, M.D. and Alan F. Schatzberg, M.D.

Department of Psychiatry
Harvard Medical School
McLean Hospital
Belmont, Massachusetts   02178

INTRODUCTION

The presence of delusions as part of the major depressive syndrome has long been recognized, but its significance for the prognosis and treatment of the depressed patient or as an important feature to discriminate a subgroup of patients has only recently been emphasized. Indeed, a growing body of evidence points toward psychotic depression being a distinct clinical entity with unique neuroendocrine and biochemical abnormalities. Particularly, considerable data have emerged that psychotic depression is characterized by pronounced increases in hypothalamic-pituitary-adrenal (HPA) axis activity. Recently, a number of observations in several species, including man, point toward glucocorticoids' increasing dopamine (DA) activity in a variety of tissues. This enhancement of dopaminergic systems by glucocorticoids has led to new hypotheses regarding the pathophysiology of psychotic depression, corticosteroid-induced psychoses in medical patients, and some of the psychiatric complications of Cushing's Disease. Data in support of these hypotheses are reviewed in this chapter.

Increased HPA Activity in Psychotic Depression

The dexamethasone suppression test (DST) has been used to explore hypothalamic-pituitary-adrenal (HPA) abnormalities in depressed patients (6). Although controversy exists as to the precise role of the DST in the evaluation of the depressed patient, there is growing agreement among many centers for specific abnormalities on the DST in psychotically depressed patients. Our group and others (7,13, 39, 41, 46, 49) have reported extremely high rates of cortisol nonsuppression after dexamethasone administration in psychotically depressed patients. In a review of six studies on the DST in psychotic depression involving 244 patients, 80 (79%) of the 101 psychotically depressed patients failed to suppress cortisol in contrast to 70 (49%) of 143 nonpsychotic depressed patients (47). Furthermore, we and others, have also reported that in patients with unipolar psychotic depression, 4 p.m. postdexamethasone cortisol levels are markedly elevated (often > 15 µg/dl) (13, 39, 49). For example, in our study (49) which included 45 unipolar (major) depressed patients, the mean ± SD 4 p.m. postdexamethasone cortisol level (13.49 ± 8.12 µg/dl) in the 14 patients with major depression with psychotic features was significantly higher than that of the 31 nonpsychotic major depressed patients (6.71 ± 4.83 µg/dl). These differences could not be attributed to age, sex, inpatient status, or recent weight loss. Moreover, 9 of the 45 patients with major depression had 4 p.m. postdexamethasone cortisol levels $\geq$ 15 µg/dl. Seven of the 9 were psychotic in contrast to 7 of 36 with 4 p.m. postdexamethasone cortisol levels < 15 µg/dl (Chi square = 11.4 p < .001). Further, all 7 patients with postdexamethasone cortisol levels $\geq$ 17 µg/dl were psychotic.

Although a high frequency of nonsuppression has been reported in patients with other affective psychoses such as mania (1), patients with nonaffective psychoses such as schizophrenia do not show as high frequencies of nonsuppression on the DST (1, 45). Specifically, we have compared our major (unipolar) and bipolar psychotic depressed patients with other groups of psychotic patients, including one containing 14 schizophrenic patients (45). The incidence of nonsuppression was significantly higher in psychotic major (unipolar) depressed patients as compared to patients with schizophrenia. Ten of 14 unipolars failed to suppress in contrast to 2 of 14 patients with schizophrenia (Fisher exact, p = .02). Moreover, all 10 unipolar nonsuppressors had 4 p.m. postdexamethasone cortisol levels > 10 µg/dl, in contrast to only one of the 14 patients with schizophrenia. Thus, psychosis by itself is not always associated with increased frequency of nonsuppression on the DST, in contrast to the interaction of unipolar depression with psychosis.

Increased corticosteroid activity, in primarily nonpsychiatric patients, has long been associated with secondary psychiatric disturbances. Exogenously administered corticosteroids are well known to produce psychiatric disturbances (depression, psychosis, or mania) in medical or psychiatric patients. Moreover, patients with conditions that are characterized by marked hypercortisolemia such as Cushing's Disease often demonstrate psychiatric disturbances (5). The extremely elevated cortisol levels seen in psychotically depressed patients have led our group to hypothesize that the development of delusions in unipolar depressed patients could in part be due to the secondary effects on monoamine activity produced by the patients own sustained hypercortisolemia (48).

Evidence for Corticosteroid Effects on Dopaminergic Systems

The effects of corticosteroids on catecholamines has been of considerable interest to researchers and clinicians over the years. Corticosteroids have been shown to have varying effects on noradrenergic systems depending on the duration of administration and the species studied (20, 51, 57, 62). The effects of corticosteroids on DA, which has been implicated in the pathophysiology of some psychotic disorders, had until recently not been studied directly--in part because unconjugated DA is normally undetectable or present in minute amounts in plasma (8, 27, 54). However, indirect data involving serum prolactin has suggested that glucocorticoids could increase DA activity. In rats, the chronic administration of dexamethasone blocks stress-induced increases in serum prolactin (12). Furthermore, in normal men, high dose cortisosteroids decrease baseline prolactin levels (9) and in patients with Cushing's Disease, or in those being treated with glucocorticoids, blunted rises in nocturnal prolactin are observed (26). Moreover, psychiatric patients and controls who suppress 4 p.m. cortisol levels below 5 µg/dl after a 1 mg dose of dexamethasone at 11 p.m. the night before also show significant decreases in serum prolactin levels (38) suggesting that corticosteroids could exert effects on dopaminergic systems (16).

More direct evidence has come from studies in a variety of animal species which point toward enhancement of dopaminergic activity by corticosteroids or corticotropin releasing factor (CRF). A single dose of dexamethasone has been shown to increase DA levels in rat carotid body (21) and DA turnover in mouse brain (23). Furthermore, methylprednisolone produces a dose related increase in DA levels in the lumbar spinal cord of cats (17) and Dunn (11) has shown that intracerebroventricularly administered CRF activates dopaminergic systems in mouse brain.

In an early experiment (44), we explored the effects of dexamethasone on the levels of unconjugated plasma DA in healthy control subjects. Dexamethasone had a significant effect on circulating unconjugated DA. Prior to dexamethasone, six of the 12 subjects had unconjugated DA detectable at 8 a.m. and only one of the 12 subjects had unconjugated DA detectable at 4 p.m. After dexamethasone, all subjects demonstrated detectable plasma unconjugated DA (Table 1).

Table 1. Effect of Dexamethasone on Unconjugated Plasma Dopamine in Man

Subject	Before Dexamethasone		After Dexamethasone	
	8:00 a.m.	4:00 p.m.	8:00 a.m.	4:00 p.m.
1	ND	ND	167	260
2	41	ND	71	187
3	ND	ND	96	75
4	102	ND	161	142
5	ND	ND	111	92
6	ND	ND	93	150
7	ND	ND	173	127
8	53	ND	42	64
9	49	63	120	195
10	ND	ND	171	176
11	54	ND	438	200
12	58	ND	213	290
Mean ± S.D.	50 ± 18	42 ± 7	155 ± 102	163 ± 70

All values are pg/ml
ND = Non-Detectable (< 40 pg/ml)

The mean plasma unconjugated DA levels after dexamethasone at 8 a.m. (155 ± 102 pg/ml) and 4 p.m. (163 ± 70 pg/ml) were significantly higher than at 8 a.m. (50 ± 18 pg/ml) and 4 p.m. (42 ± 7 pg/ml) before dexamethasone ($p < .001$).

The finding that dexamethasone administration was associated with an increase in circulating plasma DA was unexpected. The sources of DA in plasma are believed to include the central nervous system as well as several peripheral sites (28, 29, 53). Recent studies have demonstrated that most DA in plasma from normal human subjects is conjugated as sulfates or glucuronides and very little exists in the unconjugated form (22, 24, 27). The increase in plasma unconjugated DA following dexamethasone could have resulted from either a physiologically induced cellular release of DA or an alteration in the equilibrium between DA release and its metabolism by conjugation, hydroxylation, and oxidation in various organ systems.

Banki and colleagues (3) have reported that dexamethasone increases both CSF homovanillic acid (HVA) and 5-hydroxyindoleacetic acid (5-HIAA) in diverse groups of psychiatric patients, suggesting the effects of corticosteroids on dopaminergic systems could be occuring centrally. Recently, a report by Wolkowitz and colleagues (59) that a 1 mg dose of dexamethasone significantly increases plasma HVA in normal volunteers provided further evidence for a direct effect of corticosteroids on dopaminergic systems in man. However, the question still arises as to whether the effects of corticosteroids on DA systems are occuring centrally as well as peripherally. In order to address this question we proceeded to an animal model.

In our next study (43) 20 male rats of the Sprague-Dawley Strain were injected intraperitoneally at 8 a.m. with either 20 μg. (0.1cc) of dexamethasone or an equivalent volume of saline. Similarly low doses of dexamethasone have been shown to suppress corticosterone production in the rat for at least 4 hours (14) making this dose and time frame comparable to a 1 mg dexamethasone suppression test in man. Half of the saline treated group and half of the dexamethasone treated group were sacrificed at one hour and the remaining half were sacrificed at four hours after injection. Decapitation and dissection were completed within three minutes using a modification of the method of Glowinski and Iversen (15). Seven brain regions were dissected: cortex (including hippocampus) (left and right), nucleus accumbens (left and right), striatum (left and right) and hypothalamus. The concentrations of DA and 3, 4 dihydroxyphenylacetic acid (DOPAC), the major metabolite of DA in the rat, were measured using HPLC-EC. The protein content of each sample was assayed according to the Lowry method (31) and used in determining the concentration of the various monoamines and metabolites.

Dexamethasone significantly increased unconjugated DA concentration in the hypothalamus at 4 hours. In addition, an increase in DOPAC was noted, particularly at 4 hours. In the nucleus accumbens, dexamethasone significantly increased DA at both 1 and 4 hours. Similar effects on DA were not observed in the frontal cortex or striatum. In fact, DOPAC was reduced significantly at both 1 and 4 hours in both frontal cortex and striatum.

The increase in DA levels seen in the hypothalamus and nucleus accumbens after dexamethasone administration in the rat is consistent with previous reports that glucocorticoids can increase tyrosine hydroxylase (TH) activity, the rate limiting step in the biosynthesis of both DA and norepinephrine (NE). Indeed, Markey et al. (33, 34) have reported that after three days of administration, dexamethasone increased TH activity in mouse pons and locus coeruleus but not in substantia nigra. Similarly, Hanbauer and colleagues (19) have reported that dexamethasone increased TH in rat sympathetic ganglia but not in adrenal medulla and

Markey and Sze (32) have reported that TH activity in the locus coeruleus is under the regulatory influence of ACTH. The differential DA effects could also be due in part to the fact that the anatomic binding pattern of dexamethasone varies depending on the specific brain region studied (36). Thus, the increases in TH after glucocorticoid administration are highly tissue specific and could explain the differential DA effects seen in our study. Recently, Wolkowitz and colleagues (60) reported increased DA activity in the caudate of rats after subcutaneous corticosterone administration providing further evidence that glucocorticoids effect dopaminergic systems in the central nervous system.

Corticosteroid/Dopamine Hypothesis for Psychotic Depression

The direct and indirect evidence for an increase in DA activity as a result of corticosteroid administration coupled with the marked dyscontrol of the HPA axis in most patients with psychotic depression led our group to propose (48) that depressive psychosis is a secondary result of hypercortisolemia in patients who have a propensity for increasing DA activity in specific regions of brain. This corticosteroid/dopamine hypothesis does not purport to explain why patients become depressed, but rather why some depressed patients become psychotic.

To test this hypothesis in a preliminary fashion, we measured cortisol and DA in a group of psychotic depressed patients, nonpsychotic depressed patients, and normal control subjects.

METHODS

We studied 22 medication-free depressed patients (11 female and 11 male) who ranged in age from 22 to 57 years (Mean $\pm$ SD age = 37.3 $\pm$ 9.4 years). All patients were medication free at the time of the study and most were medication-free for at least two. No patient had been on neuroleptic medication for at least two weeks prior to the study. Three (1 psychotic and 2 nonpsychotic) of the 22 patients had received neuroleptics at some point in their history. One had received chlorpromazine 15 years prior, and one with psychotic depression had received perphenazine/amitriptyline one month prior. No patients had been rapidly tapered off their antidepressant medication. All patients were medically and neurologically healthy and none had a history of alcohol or drug abuse in the previous six months.

Of the 22, 16 were inpatients and 6 were outpatients at the time of the study. Patients were rated using the 21-item Hamilton Depression Rating Scale (HAM-D) (18). Mean ($\pm$ SD) HAM-D score was 21.0 $\pm$ 10.4. We included 6 less severely depressed patients (with HAM-D scores < 18) in the study because we wanted to explore the possible relationship of severity to catecholamine and cortisol levels. Using DSM-III criteria patients received the following diagnoses: major depression (N=13), dysthymic disorder (N=3), or bipolar disorder, depressed (N=6). Patients were also diagnosed using Research Diagnostic Criteria (RDC) (50). None met criteria for either Bipolar I or schizoaffective disorder (i.e., all DSM-III bipolar patients met criteria on the RDC for Bipolar II disorder). Four of the 22 patients had mood congruent psychotic features (3 women and 1 man). They ranged in age from 22 to 57 years (Mean $\pm$ SD = 45.3 $\pm$ 15.8 years).

Blood was drawn using a simple needle stick at 4 p.m. on days 1 and 2 of the study for determination of unconjugated plasma dopamine and cortisol. A 1 mg dose of dexamethasone was given at 11 p.m. on day 1 of the study.

A group of 6 healthy, medication-free control subjects (5 women and 1 man) whose ages ranged from 22 to 31 years (Mean ± SD age = 25.7 ± 3.1 years) were used as a comparison group. These 6 represent a subgroup of the 12 healthy control subjects on whom we previously reported data (44). In that study the other 6 subjects had blood drawn under different experimental conditions. In the remaining 6 subjects described below, blood samples were obtained in the identical fashion to that used in our patients.

Unconjugated plasma DA was measured using HPLC-EC methods described previously by our group (8, 44, 56). Plasma cortisol was determined by RIA methods described by our group (42, 49). Plasma cortisol and monoamine levels in the various groups were compared using one-way analysis of variance (ANOVA) and analysis of covariance (ANCOVA). Cortisol and monoamine levels were log-transformed before the ANOVA's and ANCOVA were performed because the values were not normally distributed. Post hoc analyses were performed using Student's Newman-Keuls. Data were also analyzed using Fisher Exact tests (two-tailed) and Paired t-tests.

RESULTS

Depressed Patients vs. Controls

In this study, significant differences were not observed between patients and controls in predexamethasone DA or cortisol levels. In contrast, after dexamethasone, depressed patients demonstrated higher cortisol levels (trend significance) but significantly lower DA levels (Table 2).

Table 2. Plasma Cortisol and Dopamine Levels in Normal Controls and Depressed Patients

	CONTROLS (n=6)	DEPRESSIVES (n=22)	ANOVA	
	MEAN ± S.D.	MEAN ± S.D.	F	p
PREDEXAMETHASONE				
Dopamine (pg/ml)	43.0 ± 9.8	93.0 ± 93.0	2.15	NS
Cortisol (μg/dl)	10.0 ± 5.9	12.5 ± 4.2	2.02	NS
POSTDEXAMETHASONE				
Dopamine (pg/ml)	175.3 ± 76.0	102.0 ± 90.0	4.50	.04
Cortisol (μg/dl)	1.5 ± 1.7	6.3 ± 8.0	3.37	.078

Effect of Dexamethasone on Dopamine and Cortisol

As indicated in Table 2, postdexamethasone DA in depressed patients was significantly higher than predexamethasone DA (t = 2.37, p = .03). In contrast, postdexamethasone cortisol was significantly lower than it was predexamethasone (t = 3.85, p = .001). Similarly, in control sub-

jects, postdexamethasone DA was significantly higher than predexamethasone DA (t= 4.30, p = .008) and postdexamethasone cortisol was significantly lower (t = 4.63, p = .006) than predexamethasone cortisol. Of
note, however, is that the magnitude of the increase in plasma DA in the
control subjects (~100 pg/ml) was ten times greater than the increase
seen in the patients (~10 pg/ml).

Depressive Subgroups and Controls

In this study, 7 of 22 patients (32%) failed to suppress their cortisol. A significantly higher rate of nonsuppression was observed in the
psychotic patients (4 of 4) as compared with 3 of 18 nonpsychotic patients (Fisher exact, p = .008) or 0 of 6 control subjects (Fisher exact, p = .005).

As indicated in Tables 3 and 4, one-way ANOVA with Student Newman-
Keuls revealed a number of significant differences among the nonpsychotic depressed patients, psychotic depressed patients and controls.
(Refer to Tables 3 and 4). The mean (± SD) DA levels in the psychotic
subgroup was significantly higher both pre- and postdexamethasone than
those seen in the nonpsychotic depressed patients and significantly
higher than the control group prior to dexamethasone (Tables 3 and 4).
Nonpsychotic patients had significantly lower postdexamethasone DA
levels than did the control subjects (Table 4). The psychotically depressed group had significantly higher pre- and postdexamethasone cortisol levels than the nonpsychotic depressed group or the control group.
There were no significant differences between nonpsychotic depressed
patients and control subjects on pre- or postdexamethasone cortisol
values.

To explore for possible effects of age, we performed an ANCOVA covarying for age. Diagnosis exerted a main effect on all intergroup
differences in cortisol and DA with the exception of predexamethasone
cortisol where a main effect was observed for age (F = 8.6, p = .007)
but not for diagnosis. (Age exerted a significant effect on only one
other measure - predexamethasone DA - but diagnosis also exerted a significant effect on this measure). However, the small sample sizes make
it difficult to interpret the possible effects of age on predexamethasone cortisol and DA. Further studies are needed in a larger sample to
ferret out the precise contribution of age to differences in predexamethasone cortisol and DA levels seen between psychotically depressed
patients and controls.

Distribution of Dopamine and Cortisol Levels in Psychotic
vs. Nonpsychotic Depressed Patients

All 4 psychotically depressed patients had extremely elevated predexamethasone plasma DA levels; all were ≥ 200 pg/ml. In contrast, the
highest predexamethasone DA value in the 18 nonpsychotic patients was
90 pg/ml. Similar differences in distributions were noted when the two
groups were compared on postdexamethasone DA levels.

The 4 psychotic patients also had predexamethasone cortisol levels
that were above the median point for the depressed group (14 µg/dl) in
contrast to only 6 of 18 nonpsychotic patients (Fisher exact p < .02).
While all 4 psychotically depressed patients had postdexamethasone cor-

TABLE 3

PREDEXAMETHASONE DOPAMINE AND CORTISOL LEVELS

IN DEPRESSED PATIENTS AND NORMAL CONTROLS

	NONPSYCHOTIC (N=18)	PSYCHOTIC (N=4)	CONTROLS (N=6)	ANOVA		NEWMAN-KEULS*
	MEAN ± S.D.	MEAN ± S.D.	MEAN ± S.D.	F	p	
Dopamine	50.7 ± 17.5	282.0 ± 24.8	43.0 ± 9.8	79.8	<.001	P v. NP, P v. C
Cortisol	11.2 ± 3.9	18.5 ± 3.1	10.0 ± 5.9	4.6	.02	P v. NP, P v. C

*SIGNIFICANT AT $p \leq .05$

VALUES LOG-CORRECTED PRIOR TO ANALYSIS OF VARIANCE

CORTISOL IS EXPRESSED AS µG/DL AND DOPAMINE AS PG/ML

TABLE 4

POSTDEXAMETHASONE DOPAMINE AND CORTISOL LEVELS

IN DEPRESSED PATIENTS AND NORMAL CONTROLS

	NONPSYCHOTIC (N=18)	PSYCHOTIC (N=4)	CONTROLS (N=6)	ANOVA		NEWMAN-KEULS*
	MEAN ± S.D.	MEAN ± S.D.	MEAN ± S.D.	F	p	
Dopamine	69.2 ± 30.1	278.5 ± 58.8	175.3 ± 76.0	24.5	<.001	P v. NP, NP v. C
Cortisol	3.3 ± 6.0	17.5 ± 6.8	1.5 ± 1.7	10.3	<.001	P v. NP, P v. C

*SIGNIFICANT AT p≤.05

VALUES LOG-CORRECTED PRIOR TO ANALYSIS OF VARIANCE

CORTISOL IS EXPRESSED AS µG/DL AND DOPAMINE AS PG/ML

tisol levels > 10 μg/dl, only 2 of 18 nonpsychotic depressed patients
had similarly high postdexamethasone cortisol values (Fisher exact
p < .01).

Cortisol and Dopamine vs.Severity

Given that we included a few nonpsychotic patients with either dysthymic disorder or milder major depressions, we explored the effect of
severity of depression on DA and cortisol values by comparing psychotic
and nonpsychotic depressed patients using ANCOVA, covarying for HAM-D
scores. Significant main effects for diagnosis (i.e., psychosis) were
still observed on predexamethasone DA (F= 104.8, p < .001), predexamethasone cortisol (F = 6.4, p = .02), postdexamethasone DA (F = 29.6, p <
.001), and postdexamethasone cortisol (F = 8.2, p = .01). HAM-D also
exerted a significant effect on predexamethasone DA (F = 32.1, p < .001),
postdexamethasone DA (F = 11.7, p = .003) and postdexamethasone cortisol
(F = 5.6, p = .03) but not on predexamethasone cortisol. In addition,
we further assessed the possible effect of severity by dividing the
nonpsychotic patients by HAM-D score (< or ≥ 18). Specifically, nonpsychotic patients with HAM-D scores ≥ 18 had significantly lower (F =
5.00, p = .04) predexamethasone DA levels (44.6 ± 9.5 pg/ml) than patients with HAM-D scores < 18 (63.0 ± 23.8 pg/ml). No significant differences in postdexamethasone DA or pre- and postdexamethasone cortisol
levels were found when the nonpsychotic group was divided by HAM-D
score. These data all suggest that the elevated predexamethasone DA
levels in the psychotically depressed group cannot be explained solely
on the basis of greater severity. However, further studies on larger
samples will be needed to determine the possible contribution of severity to differences in DA or cortisol levels.
    In this study of depressed patients dexamethasone again appeared to
increase DA levels but to much lesser extent than the normal controls.
In addition, more severely depressed nonpsychotic patients had significantly lower predexamethasone unconjugated DA levels when compared
with less severely depressed patients. These findings are consistent
with recent reports (59, 61) that a 1 mg dose of dexamethasone elevates plasma HVA in normal controls but may lower it in depressed patients. It is also possible that the potential for further enhancement of DA levels has already been exhaused by a chronic hypercortisolemic state or that increased levels of circulating cortisol has resulted in a blunted response to dexamethasone. Moreover, a relative
blunting of the DA response to dexamethasone in depressed patients is
consistent with the observation by Judd and colleagues (25) that depressed patients have lower mean basal prolactin levels and exhibit
blunted prolactin responses to methadone when compared with normal controls or nondepressed psychiatric patients.

DISCUSSION

The above studies indicate that psychotically depressed patients have
significantly higher pre- and postdexamethasone cortisol, as well as
higher pre- and postdexamethasone DA than nonpsychotic depressed patients. The higher cortisol levels seen in the patients with psychotic

depression as compared to nonpsychotic depressed patients are consistent with previous studies by our group and others. In addition, psychotically depressed patients demonstrated significantly higher pre- and postdexamethasone cortisol and higher predexamethasone DA levels than did the normal control subjects.

In this study only patients with psychotic depression demonstrated markedly elevated plasma unconjugated DA levels ($\geq$ 200 pg/ml) both pre- and postdexamethasone. However, the observation that some depressed patients with predexamethasone cortisol levels $\geq$ 14 µg/dl demonstrated neither DA levels $\geq$ 200 pg/ml or psychosis indicates that there may be particular risk factors for developing pronounced increases in DA levels such as increased tyrosine hydroxylase (TH) activity or decreased dopamine-B-hydroxylase (DBH) activity.

The finding of elevated pre- and postdexamethasone plasma DA levels are consistent with a number of recent studies on psychotic depression. Psychotically depressed patients have been reported (52) to have significantly higher CSF HVA levels than their nonpsychotic counterparts. Another study indicated that increasing CSF HVA levels occurring with antidepressant treatment were associated with emergent psychosis and that clinical response to lithium carbonate added to an antidepressant treatment in agitated, psychotic depressed patients was accompanied by significant decreases in CSF HVA levels (30). However, caution must be exercised in interpreting CSF HVA levels in depression because they may be derived primarily from basal ganglion (40) and may also be correlated with relative agitation or retardation (55). The present study is also consistent with recent reports that depressed females with psychosis exhibit higher plasma HVA levels than do healthy female control subjects (10) and that psychotically depressed patients have elevated CSF HVA levels (2).

Although the exact mechanism by which DA levels become elevated in psychotic depression remains for future research, there is currently evidence that glucocorticoids can produce increases in DA synthesis by increasing TH activity as was described earlier. Another possible factor is relatively decreased DBH activity. Low DBH levels have been reported in the serum of psychotically depressed patients but not normal controls (37). In contrast, nonpsychotic depressed patients have been reported to have significantly higher serum DBH than controls (35). However, it is unlikely that DBH could be the sole explanation for the elevated DA levels since it is a trait dependent marker and has been reported to not normalize with improvement (37). Yet it is conceivable that decreased activity of DBH may represent a biologic vulnerability for the development of psychotic depression by allowing increased DA levels in the context of increased DA synthesis. Since DBH and TH have been shown to be under strong genetic control in various species (4, 58) and since the susceptibility of other catecholamine enzymes to "induction" by corticosteroids is also under genetic influence (4), they could be important clues to a relative vulnerability for the development of psychotic depression or steroid-induced psychoses.

In summary, considerable data have emerged that point to close relationships among psychotic depression, high DA levels, and high cortisol levels, suggesting that high DA and cortisol levels could account for the development of delusions in the context of a depressive episode, other affective psychotic states, and corticosteroid-induced psychoses. Further studies in larger samples of patients are needed and are underway to replicate our findings and to explore the possible role of DBH as a risk factor and differences in plasma levels of HVA, a key DA metabolite. Moreover, the specific roles of cortisol, ACTH, and CRF as enhancers of dopaminergic activity need to be elucidated, particularly in their possible mediation of psychotic thinking in depressed patients.

REFERENCES

1. Arana, G.W., Barreira, P.J., Cohen, B.M., Lipinski, J.F., Fogelson, D. (1983): Am. J. Psychiatry, 140:1521.
2. Asberg-Wistedt, A., Wistedt, B., Bertilsson, L. (1985): Arch. Gen. Psychiatry, 42:925.
3. Banki, C.M., Arato, M., Papp, A. (1983): Biol. Psychiatry, 18:1033.
4. Barchas: J.D., Ciarennello: R.D., Kessler: S., Hamburg: D.A. (1975): In: Genetic Research in Psychiatry, edited by R.R. Fieve, D. Rosenthal, H. Brill, pp. 27-62. The Johns Hopkins University Press, Baltimore.
5. Carpenter, W.T., Gruen, P.H. (1982): J. Clin. Psychopharmacol 2:91.
6. Carroll, B.J., Feinberg, M., Greden, J.F., Tarika, J., Albala, A. A., Haskett, R.E., James, N., Kronfol, Z., Lohr, N., Steiner, M., DeVigne, J.P., Young, E. (1981): Arch. Gen. Psychiatry, 38:15.
7. Carroll, B.J., Greden, J.F., Feinberg, M., James, N., Haskett, R. F., Steiner, M., Tarika, J. (1980): Psychiatry Res., 2:251.
8. Causon, R.L., Carruthers, M.E., Rodnight, R. (1981): Annal. Biochem., 116:223.
9. Copinschi, G., L'Hermite, M., LeClercq, R., Goldstein, J., Vanhaelst, L., Virasoro, E., Robyn, C. (1975): J. Clin. Endocrinol Metab., 40:442.
10. Devanand, D.P., Bowers, M.B., Hoffman, F.J., Nelson, J.C. (1985): Psychiatry Res., 15:1
11. Dunn, A.J. (1985): J. Neurochem. Abstr., 44:S.97.
12. Euker, J.S., Meites, J., Riegle, G.D. (1975): Endocrinology, 96:85.
13. Evans, D.L., Burnett, G.B., Nemeroff, C.B. (1983): Am. J. Psychiatry, 140:586.
14. Feldman, S., Conforti, N. (1976): Endocrinology, 82:785.
15. Glowinski, J., Iversen, L.L. (1966): J. Neurochem., 13:655.
16. Gruen, P.H., Sachar, E.J., Langer, G., Altman, N., Leifer, M., Frantz, A., Halpern, F.S. (1978): Arch. Gen. Psychiatry, 35:108.
17. Hall, E.D., McGinley, P.A. (1982): J. Neurochem., 38:1787.
18. Hamilton, M. (1960): J. Neurol. Neurosurg. Psychiatry, 23:56.
19. Hanbauer, I., Guidotti, A., Costa, E. (1975): Brain Res., 85:527.
20. Harrison, T.S., Chawla, R.C., Wojtalik, R.S. (1968): New Engl. J. Med., 279:136.
21. Hellstrom S., Commissiony, J., Hanbauer, I. (1979): Neuroscience, 4:1157.
22. Imai, K., Suguira, M., and Tamura, Z. (1970): Chem. Pharm. Bull., 18:2134.
23. Iuvone, P.M., Morasco, J., Dunn, A.J. (1977): Brain Res., 120:571.
24. Johnson, G.A., Baker, C.A., Smith, R.T. (1980): Life Sci., 26:1591.
25. Judd, L.L., Risch, C., Parker, D.C., Janowsky, D.S., Segal, D.S., Huey, L.Y. (1982): Arch. Gen. Psychiatry, 39:1413.

26. Krieger, D.T., Howanitz, P.J., Frantz, A.G. (1976): J. Clin. Endocrinol. Metab., 42:260.
27. Kuchel, O., Buu, N.T., Unger, T., Lis, M. (1979): J. Clin. Endocrinol. Metab., 48:425.
28. Lackovic, Z., Neff, N.H. (1983): Life Sci., 32:1665.
29. Levin, B.E., Hubschmann, O.R. (1980): Neurology 30:65.
30. Linnoila, M., Karoum, F., Potter, W.Z. (1983): Arch. Gen. Psychiatry, 40:1015.
31. Lowry, O.H., Rosebrough, N.J., Farr, A.L., Randall, R.J. (1951): J. Biol. Chem., 193:265.
32. Markey, K.A., Sze, P.Y. (1984): Neuroendocrinology, 38:269.
33. Markey, K.A., Towle, A.C., Sze, P.Y. (1980): Abstracts of the Society of Neuroscience, 6:53.27.
34. Markey, K.A., Towle, A.C., Sze, P.Y. (1982): Endocrinology, 111:1519.
35. Matuzas, W., Meltzer, H.Y., Uhlenhuth, E.H., Glass, R.M., Tong, C. (1982): Biol. Psychiatry, 17:1415.
36. McEwen, B.S. (1980): Psychoneuroendocrinol, 5:1.
37. Meltzer, H.Y., Cho, H.W., Carroll, B.J., Russo, P. (1976): Arch. Gen. Psychiatry, 33:585.
38. Meltzer, H.Y., Fang, V.S., Tricou, B.J., Roberston, A., Pikaya, S.K. (1982): Am. J. Psychiatry, 139:763.
39. Mendlewicz, J., Charles, G., Franckson, J.M. (1982): Br. J. Psychiatry, 141:464.
40. Post, R.M., Goodwin, F.K. (1975): Science, 190:488.
41. Rhimer, Z., Arato, M., Szadoczky, E., Revai, K., Demeter E., Gyorgy, S., Udvarhelyi, P. (1984): Br. J. Psychiatry, 145:508.
42. Rosenbaum, A.H., Schatzberg, A.F., MacLaughlin, R.A., Synder, K., Jiang, N.S., Istrup, D., Rothschild, A.J., Klineman, B. (1984): Am. J. Psychiatry, 141:1550.
43. Rothschild, A.J., Langlais, P.J., Schatzberg, A.F., Miller, M.M., Salomon, M.S., Lerbinger, J.E., Cole, J.O., Bird, E.D. (1985): Life Sci., 36:2491.
44. Rothschild, A.J., Langlais, P.J., Schatzberg, A.F., Walsh, F.X., Cole, J.O., Bird, E.D. (1984): J. Psychiatric Res., 18:217.
45. Rothschild, A.J., Schatzberg, A.F., Rosenbaum, A.H., Stahl, J.B., Cole, J.O. (1982): Br. J. Psychiatry, 141:471.
46. Rudorfer, M.V., Hwu, H.G., Clayton, P.J. (1982): Biol. Psychiatry, 17:41.
47. Schatzberg, A.F., Rothschild, A.J., Bond, T.C., Cole, J.O. (1984): Psychopharm. Bull., 20:362.
48. Schatzberg, A.F., Rothschild, A.J., Langlais, P.J., Bird, E.D., Cole, J.O. (1985): J. Psychiatric Res., 19:57.
49. Schatzberg, A.F., Rothschild, A.J., Stahl, J.B., Bond, T.C., Rosenbaum, A.H., Lofgren, S.B., MacLaughlin, R.A., Sullivan, M.A., Cole, J.O. (1983): Am. J. Psychiatry, 140:88.
50. Spitzer, R.L., Endicott, J., Robins, E. (1978): Arch. Gen. Psychiatry, 35:773.
51. Stene, M., Panagiotis, N., Tuck, M.L., Sowers, J.R., Mayes, D., Berg, G. (1980): J. Clin. Endocrinol. Metab., 51:1340.
52. Sweeney, D., Nelson, C., Bowers, M., Maas, J., Heninger, G. (1978): Lancet, 2:100.
53. Thorner, M.O. (1975): Lancet, 1:662.
54. Van Loon, G.R., Schwartz, L., Sole, M.J. (1979): Life Sci., 24:2273

55. Van Praag, H.M., Korf, J., Lakke, J.O.W.F., Schut, T (1975): Psychological Med., 5:138.

56. Walsh, F.X., Langlais, P.J., Bird, E.D. (1982): Clin. Chem. 28: 382.

57. Wiechman, B.E., Borowitz, J.L. (1979): Pharmacology, 18:195.

58. Winter, H., Herschel, M., Propping. P., Friedl, W., Vogel, F. (1978): Psychopharmacology, 57:63.

59. Wolkowitz, O.M., Sutton, M.E., Doran, A.R., Labarca, R., Roy, A., Thomas, J.W., Pickar, D., Paul, S.M. (1985): Psychiatry Res., 16:101.

60. Wolkowitz, O.M., Sutton, M., Koulu, M., Labarca, R., Wilkinson, L., Doran, A., Hauger, R., Pickar, D., Cawley, J. (1986): Eur. J. Pharmacology 122:329.

61. Wolkowitz, O.M., Sutton, M.E., Labarca R., Roy, A., Doran, A.R., Goodwin, F.D., Paul, S.M. (1984): Presented at the 23rd Annual Meeting of the American College of Neuropsychopharmacology, San Juan, Puerto Rico, December 10-14.

62. Wurtman, R., Axelrod, J. (1966): J. Biol. Chem., 241:2301.

ACKNOWLEDGEMENTS

The authors were supported in part by Grant No. MH-38671 from the National Institute of Mental Health, a grant from the Engelhard Foundation, and a private grant to support the Depression Research Facility. We are grateful to Patti Mancuso and Nancy Lucero for preparation of the manuscript.

Subject Index